CREATINE
Nature's Muscle Builder

RAY SAHELIAN, M.D.
DAVE TUTTLE

Avery Publishing Group
Garden City Park, New York

The author, publisher, endorsers, distributors, researchers, or anyone else whose name appears in this book shall have neither liability, nor responsibility, to anyone with respect to any loss or damage caused, or alleged to be caused, directly or indirectly by the information contained in this book. Should you have any questions or concerns about using creatine, the authors and publisher strongly suggest consulting your physician.

Photos on pages 23, 25, 29, 65, 81, 113, supplied with permission of Jim Amentler; photos on pages 15, 38, 67, 71, 77, 99, 103 supplied with permission of Photodisc; photo on page 35 supplied with permission of Jason Mathas; cover photo supplied with permission of Mike Neveux.

Cover design and typesetting: William Gonzalez
Illustrations: Russell Kurtz
In-house editor: Jennifer Santo
Printer: Paragon Press, Honesdale, PA

Library of Congress Cataloging-in-Publication Data

Sahelian, Ray
    Creatine: Nature's Muscle Builder / Ray Sahelian and Dave Tuttle.
    p. cm.
    Includes bibliographical references and index.
    Preassigned LCCN: 96-84272
    ISBN 0-89529-777-9
                        / 3 ²

    1. Creatine kinase.   I. Tuttle, Dave.   II. Title.
    QP606.C73S34 1997   615.773 574.192'5
                                QBI96-40368

Printed in the United States of America

10   9

CONTENTS

ACKNOWLEDGEMENTS

We wish to thank Conrad P. Earnest, Ph.D., and Dr. Rick Kreider for their cooperation in providing reference material.

We also wish to thank the men and women who participated in our survey. In addition to those who are profiled in the book and the many who want to remain anonymous, we appreciate the contributions of the following: Michael Alexis, Sean Allen, John Appleby, Armand Azurdia, Roehl Barreras, Martin Bean, Scott Brandin, Raymond Campisi, John Defendis, Mark Frey, Vince Galanti, Patrick Hopkins, David Jennings, Kevin Lewis, Michael Meehan, Todd Micletti, George Mihalopoulos, Dr. Max More, Donny O'Hearn, Ray Owen, Glenn Parker, Juan Perez, Dr. Christopher Sabatino, Richard Shapiro, Brian Shiers, Kirk Sullivan, and Roger Williams.

PREFACE

We're excited to share with you the benefits we have discovered about a nutrient that will, without a doubt, become very popular. *Creatine: Nature's Muscle Builder* is the first book that discusses this fascinating supplement in depth. We have evaluated decades of research, reviewed hundreds of articles, interviewed top researchers involved in the field, and gathered personal stories of creatine users to give you all the practical information you need to use this nutrient wisely and efficiently. We feel that creatine can be beneficial to men and women in all age groups who want to build muscle and look their best.

Athletes are always looking for ways to boost their strength, lift more weight, or sprint faster. Even a small improvement can give them a competitive edge that can be a deciding factor in winning a race or taking home the trophy. Bodybuilders, wrestlers, and football players also know that increased strength can lead to greater muscle mass, which can help them dominate their opponents on the playing field.

Athletes have been taking performance enhancers for a long time. These so-called ergogenic aids can sometimes make a dramatic difference in an athlete's ability to excel, and give him or her a needed edge in today's super-competitive sport scene. Unfortunately, not everything that is promoted as an ergogenic aid is effective. Some, in fact, are useless, while others can make a significant difference in strength, muscle size, and performance. Creatine is one of the winners.

We would like to make it clear that we did not receive financial support from any vitamin company or creatine manufacturer, distributor, or retailer while writing this book. We recognized that sponsorship by a group with vested interests in promoting creatine would make our conclusions suspect. As a result, we decided to write this book independently, in order to give you, the consumer, all of the facts without any of the commercials or promotional hype. Our objective is to provide you with accurate information. It will then be up to you, in consultation with your health care provider or trainer, to determine whether creatine is appropriate for your unique circumstance.

Ray Sahelian, M.D.

Dave Tuttle

CHAPTER 1

THE ABCs OF CREATINE

Whether you're young or old, male or female, an accomplished athlete or someone who has just started an exercise program, you need to know about creatine. Many supplements touted over the years as performance enhancers have come and gone, but creatine is here to stay. It has become the most popular muscle-building nutrient ever sold. Why? Because it works. Yes, it *really* works.

What Is Creatine?

When we told our friends that we were writing a book on creatine, some of them had quizzical responses. "You're writing on creating? Creating what?" "Is it an herb?"

Creatine (pronounced krē'ə tēn') is a nutrient that is naturally found in our bodies. It is made from a combination of the three amino acids: arginine, glycine, and methionine (see page 5). Creatine helps provide the energy our muscles need to move, particularly movements

1

which are quick and explosive in nature. This includes the types of motions involved in most sports. Approximately 95 percent of the body's creatine supply is found in the skeletal muscles. The remaining 5 percent is scattered throughout the rest of the body, with the highest concentrations in the heart, brain, and testes. (Sperm is chock-full of creatine!)

The human body gets most of the creatine it needs from food or dietary supplements. Creatine is easily absorbed from the intestinal tract into the bloodstream. When dietary consumption is inadequate to meet the body's needs, a limited supply can be synthesized from the amino acids arginine, glycine, and methionine. This production occurs in the liver, pancreas, and kidneys.

What Does Creatine Do?

There are at least three different ways that creatine is thought to have an ergogenic effect.

• *Increases the volume of muscle cells*

Soon after you begin using creatine, you will feel your muscles getting larger and harder. This is due to an increase in the quantity of fluid stored inside your muscle cells. As the amount of this intracellular fluid rises, it pushes against the cell membrane and actually expands the cell's volume. The microscopic boost in mass, multiplied by the millions of muscle cells, results in bigger and more shapely muscles. This process is technically known as volumization.

• *Serves as an energy reservoir*

Creatine exists in two different forms within the muscle fiber: as free (chemically-unbound) creatine and as creatine phosphate. This latter form of creatine makes up two-thirds of the total creatine supply. When your muscles contract, the initial fuel for this movement is a compound called ATP. Unfortunately, there is only enough ATP to provide energy for less than 10 seconds, so for muscle contraction to continue, more ATP must be produced. Creatine phosphate comes to the rescue by giving up part of its molecule to recreate ATP. This ATP can then be "burned" again as fuel for more muscle contraction.

The bottom line is that your ability to regenerate ATP depends on your supply of creatine. The more creatine in your muscle cells, the more ATP can be remade, and the easier it is to train your muscles to their maximum potential. It's that simple. This greater ATP resynthesis also keeps your body from relying on another energy system called glycolysis, which has lactic acid as a by-product. This lactic acid creates the burning sensation you feel during intense exercise. But if you keep on using ATP because of all the creatine you have, you can minimize the amount of lactic acid produced and actually exercise longer and harder. This helps you gain strength, power, and muscle size. You won't get fatigued as easily, either.

• *Enhances protein synthesis*

Creatine is also thought to enhance your body's ability to make proteins within muscle fibers. Two of these proteins, actin and myosin, are essential to all muscle contraction. So when you build up your supply of these contractile proteins, you actually increase your muscle's ability to perform physical work. And the more work you do (whether it's lifting weights or swimming 100-meter sprints), the stronger you become over time.

How Much Creatine Is in My Body?

The amount of creatine you have in your body depends mostly on the amount of muscle you have. (There is no creatine in body fat.) The average 155 pound (70 kilogram) person has a total of about 120 grams (4.2 ounces) of creatine in his or her body at any one time. Vegetarians, by and large, have lower creatine levels than meateaters. A 1979 study by Walker showed that the average sedentary person uses up about 2 grams of creatine per day. This creatine is broken down into a waste product called creatinine, which is collected by the kidneys and excreted in the urine. Athletes use up much more than 2 grams per day, with the exact amount depending on the type of sport, the intensity level, and the individual's muscle mass.

Can I Get Enough Creatine From My Diet?

The average person consumes about one gram of creatine per day. Creatine is found in moderate amounts in the skeletal muscle of most meats and fish. Good sources of dietary creatine include tuna, cod, salmon, herring, beef, and pork. Tiny amounts are found in milk and even cranberries. While it would seem logical that chicken and turkey have creatine as well, we were unable to find any published data to confirm this. Cooking destroys part of the creatine that exists in these foods.

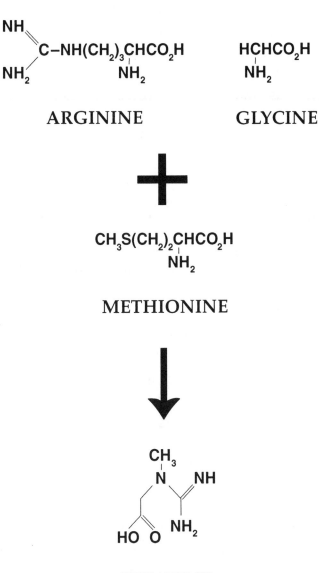

ARGININE　　　**GLYCINE**

METHIONINE

CREATINE

Creatine is formed from a combination of three amino acids.

An important thing to remember is that meats and fish have relatively high amounts of cholesterol. Most meats, especially beef and pork, also contain high quantities of fat. This fat and cholesterol can contribute to cardiovascular diseases, so it's best to avoid eating large amounts of these foods. A better solution is the non-fat, no-cholesterol supplement called creatine monohydrate.

Is Creatine Something New That Scientists Have Discovered?

While researching the scientific information published about this nutrient, we were surprised to learn that creatine was first discovered in 1832 by the French scientist Chevreul. This was way before barbells were invented! Creatine was first found in meats, and later, in 1847, a sharp observer noticed that the meat from foxes killed in the wild had ten times as much creatine as the meat from inactive, domesticated foxes. He concluded that creatine accumulates in muscles as a consequence of physical activity.

In the early 20th century, it was discovered that not all of the creatine consumed by humans is excreted in the urine. This led to the recognition that creatine is, in fact, stored within the body. In 1912, researchers found that ingesting creatine can dramatically boost the creatine content of muscle. Then, in 1927, they discovered creatine phosphate, and determined that creatine is a key player in the metabolism of skeletal muscle (Greenhaff, 1995).

There have been literally thousands of studies published on creatine. However, most of the studies focusing on creatine and sports performance have been done since the early 1990s. It is these studies that we will focus on in this book.

Who Can Benefit From Creatine?

Anyone, of any age, has the potential to benefit from creatine. If you want to be stronger, have more muscle mass, or just feel better about your body, creatine can help. Although the research on creatine and exercise performance is relatively new, it appears that the greatest benefits occur in those sports which involve short, intense bursts of energy. That is because these sports rely most heavily on ATP as an energy source. Athletes in bodybuilding, powerlifting, martial arts, sprinting, and track and field events such as javelin and shot-put will greatly benefit due to greater strength. So will wrestlers, swimmers, football, hockey, basketball, and tennis players. We doubt that creatine will be of any benefit for people who comfortably cruise on a cart around the golf course and occasionally get up to putt. Other sports where creatine is not likely to be of any significant benefit include bowling, skeet shooting, and certainly billiards.

It is still unclear whether athletes involved in endurance activities, such as marathon running or long-distance bicycling, will benefit from creatine supplementation. Stroud mentioned anecdotal reports that people in these sports may benefit, although other evidence shows that creatine either does not help or may actually be counterproductive. The difficulty in these situations appears to center on the increased muscle mass which creatine provides. While it's great if you're a bodybuilder or wrestler, it can be a detriment if you have to carry all that weight around during a marathon or triathlon. In such cases, there is a tradeoff between the increased strength you get from creatine and the increased muscle mass. Further research will provide us with more definitive answers as to what role creatine can play in endurance-type sports.

90 And Still Pumping?

Older individuals with decreased muscle mass could also benefit from creatine supplementation. Since creatine boosts strength and protein synthesis, it should help to reduce the muscle wasting that can occur with disease and the aging process. A new study by Earnest shows that creatine can reduce cholesterol and lipid levels in the blood, as well, which would be a major health benefit for everyone.

Being more muscular can also lead to an improved sense of self-esteem and well-being. Older individuals can look and feel years younger. Stronger muscles will lead to fewer falls and bone fractures, too. The quick gains that creatine provides will also motivate users to continue exercising. We know that exercising leads to stronger bones and a healthier heart. Therefore, even though creatine is technically not an anti-aging nutrient, it indirectly can lead to life span extension by encouraging people to exercise more. Creatine will help a large segment of the population to become more physically fit, improving their long-term quality of life.

Is Creatine Safe?

Experiments with the administration of creatine to humans have been going on for over a century. Dr. Paul

Balsom of the Karolinska Institute in Stockholm, Sweden, is one of the world's leading experts on creatine. In a review article published in 1994 in *Sports Medicine*, he states that "to the best of our knowledge, the only documented adverse effect that has been associated with creatine supplementation is an increase in body mass."

We suspect that most users will gladly accept this "adverse effect."

One caution we'd like to make is that the studies that used high dosages of creatine, such as 20 grams per day, were only a month or less in duration. As a result, we do not have controlled, scientific studies which indicate exactly what happens to users taking large amounts of creatine for many months or even years. The only studies that have involved long-term supplementation used dosages of 8 grams or less per day. These studies showed that creatine is effective in treating gyrate atrophy (an eye disease) and GAMT deficiency (which can impair development of motor function in infants). These and other health benefits of creatine are discussed in Chapter 7. So far, there are no long-term studies on athletes and sports performance.

As part of our research for this book, we distributed a detailed survey to athletes in three states. Personal interviews with men and women who have used creatine for over a year did not reveal any long-term side effects about which you should be concerned. Nor is there a particular reason to think that there should be a problem, given the way in which creatine is synthesized and excreted by the body. Minor side effects mentioned included diarrhea and nausea, which some users said occurred when they took dosages greater than those recommended in this book. These symptoms went away when the dosage was reduced.

Is It Legal To Use Creatine During Competition?

At the time of the printing of this book, the International Olympic Committee had not put creatine on its list of banned substances. This may be because it is a dietary component of most meats and fish, so it is difficult to distinguish who is taking oral creatine supplements and who is just eating more meat. This situation is unlikely to change, so we are predicting an explosion of creatine use at all athletic events, including the Olympics, in the coming years.

For example, an article appearing in the *San Diego Union-Tribune* on October 20, 1996, entitled "Creatine Supplement From Beef Is Worth Getting Pumped About," quotes Michael Barnes, Strength Development Coordinator for the San Francisco 49ers, as saying that at least 75 percent of his players are on this supplement.

Can I Build Muscle With Creatine Even if I Don't Work Out?

You will gain some lean mass as you increase the amount of creatine stored in your muscles, since creatine augments the muscles' water content, expanding their volume. But if you don't do any athletic training, your gains will be far less than they could be with a combined program of creatine supplementation and exercise.

CHAPTER 2

THE PROOF IS IN
THE POWDER

For a number of years I've been looking for a supplement that could bulk me up. I'm a powerlifter, and so far I've stayed away from anabolic steroids. I first heard about creatine six months ago from a friend who thought highly of it. I was skeptical, since, throughout the years that I've been involved in weight training, a lot of supplements have been hyped as ideal muscle builders.

My friend kept persisting. She kept telling me that this stuff had really benefited her. Knowing that she didn't sell the product, and had no monetary incentive to recommend it, I finally decided to give it a try. It didn't take long to make me a believer.

Before I continue taking creatine for a long time, though, I'm wondering how much research has actually been done on this nutrient?
— Stan S., age 30, Brooklyn, NY

Scientists have researched creatine for over a century, but the specific relationship between creatine supplementation and athletic performance wasn't really explored until the early 1990s. Since that time, dozens of studies have been completed around the world which show the effectiveness of creatine in a variety of situations. In this chapter we will review seven of these studies.

The Pioneer Study on Creatine

The first study that gave us a good idea of how well creatine is absorbed and metabolized was back in 1992. Dr. Roger Harris and colleagues from the Karolinska Institute in Stockholm, Sweden, wanted to test whether oral administration of creatine would increase the amount of creatine in blood and muscles. They found that the blood level of creatine increased only slightly when they gave their subjects 1 gram of creatine monohydrate (the stable form of creatine that all supplements are made of). However, when the study participants received 5 grams, there was a significant rise in their creatine blood levels.

Over the next few days, the researchers gave 5 grams of creatine monohydrate four to six times per day to seventeen volunteers, and found a significant increase in the creatine content of a thigh muscle (quadriceps femoris). In some, the increase was as much as 50 percent.

Would there be a difference in the creatine content of muscles with exercise? A simple way to find out would be to exercise one leg and compare it to the leg that remained idle. Dr. Harris did just that. When one leg was exercised for one hour a day, its average creatine content was 54 percent higher than the leg that wasn't exercised. However, even the leg that wasn't exercised had a higher creatine content than it had before supplementation.

Increase in Peak Torque

In 1993, Paul Greenhaff and his associates at the Karolinska Institute conducted an experiment to measure the impact of creatine supplementation on peak torque. Torque is a measurement of the force exerted at a distance from the body. In this case, test subjects did five sets of knee extensions on a leg-extension machine. Torque always declines over time as the muscles become fatigued. Greenhaff discovered, however, that 20 grams of creatine per day significantly reduced the decline in peak torque on three of the five sets, with an average 5 percent increase in force production. The improvement was near significance on the other two sets. This experiment showed that creatine helps you stay stronger for a longer period of time, allowing you to generate more force.

There was also a significant drop in the blood level of ammonia, a toxic by-product created when ATP stores are low. This indicates that the greater availability of creatine permitted more ATP turnover and prevented the formation of unwanted ammonia.

More Work Output

1993 was a busy year for the folks at the Karolinska Institute. P.D. Balsom and four of his colleagues did a study to evaluate how creatine impacts the output of work during dynamic, high-intensity, intermittent exercise. They compared the performance of test subjects during ten 6-second bouts of high-intensity cycling at two different exercise intensities. They discovered that creatine increased the work output in both cases, compared to persons using a placebo (inert substitute). The researchers also found that lactic-acid concentrations in the blood decreased, showing that relatively less energy was produced through the burning of glucose and glycogen in muscles. They also found less hypoxanthine, which is another by-product created when ATP isn't resynthesized quickly enough.

Additionally, Balsom discovered that the study participants using creatine had dramatic gains in body mass. The average increase was 2.4 pounds (1.1 kilograms) in one month. The eighteen individuals in the study had growth ranging from 0.7 pounds (0.3 kilograms) to 5.5 pounds (2.5 kilograms). Balsom attributes the improvements in performance and body weight to the higher initial availability of creatine phosphate within the muscles, and the resulting ability to maintain higher levels of ATP synthesis.

Boost in Mean Power Output

In 1994, three scientists from the University of Nottingham Medical School in England tested the effects of creatine supplementation on performance and on blood-ammonia and lactic-acid accumulations. Birch, Noble, and Greenhaff gave 5 grams of creatine four times per day to fourteen young males, who then performed three 30-second bouts of maximal cycling with four-minute rest periods in between. The results were compared with a group that got a placebo. Creatine supplementation boosted mean power output—the average amount of work accomplished per unit of time—by 6 percent during the first and second bouts of heavy exercise, although there was no improvement in the third bout. There was no observed difference between the plasma levels of lactic acid for the creatine and placebo groups, which contra-

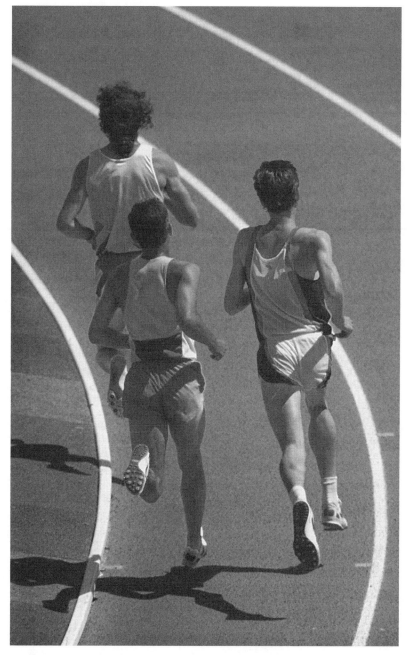

Sprinters find that creatine boosts their speed while improving their endurance.

dicted earlier findings. Those on creatine did have 19 percent less ammonia in their blood, however, despite the fact that they performed 6 percent more work than those using the placebo.

Effect of Creatine on Steady-State Exercise

At the same time, Michael Stroud and his colleagues at the University of Nottingham were researching the impact of creatine on more prolonged, submaximal exercise, also known as steady-state exercise. Eight men were given 20 grams of creatine per day for a period of five days. The researchers then took a variety of measurements during and after seven sets of treadmill exercise, at workloads ranging from 50 to 90 percent of the subjects' maximal oxygen uptake. Each set was six minutes in length. Stroud found that creatine supplementation did not have a significant effect on heart rate, oxygen consumption, blood-lactate concentration, respiratory exchange ratio, expired gas volume, or carbon dioxide production. These results have led some scientists to conclude that creatine is not an effective performance enhancer for endurance events requiring long periods of submaximal effort.

Growth in Muscular Strength, Endurance, and Bodyweight

In 1995, C.P. Earnest and his associates at Texas Women's University, University of Texas Southwestern Medical Center, and The Cooper Clinic in Dallas, Texas, conducted an experiment to see how creatine monohydrate would boost strength and endurance. They gave eight weight-trained men 20 grams of creatine per day for 28 days. The researchers also did before-and-after measurements for total body weight, the percentage of body fat, and the one-rep-maximum on the bench press (the maximum amount of weight an individual can lift and only do one repetition, or 1RM).

Earnest found that the average weight his test subjects could lift on the 1RM rose by 8.2 kilograms, a gain of over 18 pounds. That's a 6.5 percent improvement in one month. The average number of repetitions the participants could do when they lifted a weight that was only 70 percent of their 1RM also rose, from eleven to fifteen. Here was clear proof that creatine not only makes you stronger, but allows you to work longer and more intensely as well.

The researchers also discovered that there was a 3.7 pound (1.7 kilogram) increase in total body weight with only a 0.2 pound (0.1 kilogram) increase in body fat. This is a 2 percent gain in the athletes' average lean muscle mass within thirty days. The researchers concluded that "these results demonstrate the efficacy of creatine monohydrate as an ergogenic aid. The ability to perform greater muscular work, per given work task, provides a greater muscular overload that may promote an increased adaptive response in muscular structure and function." This means that creatine allows you to perform more work, stimulating increased muscle growth.

Differences Between Fixed-Intensity and Maximal Exercise

In 1995, P.D. Balsom and colleagues at the Karolinska Institute did another study on creatine. Seven men were asked to perform repeated bouts of exercise on a cycle ergometer—which measures the amount of work done by a muscle—both before and after six days of creatine supplementation. The dose was 20 grams of creatine monohydrate per day. These volunteers did five bouts of a fixed-intensity workout lasting six seconds, each followed by a thirty-second recovery period. This was followed forty seconds later by one ten-second maximal workout. Jump performance was also measured during this second phase. Samples of muscle tissue were extracted from a leg muscle (vastus lateralis) to evaluate its creatine content and other parameters.

Balsom found that supplementation boosted the total amount of creatine in muscle (free creatine plus creatine phosphate) by 18 percent before the test subjects began exercising. After the first five bouts of fixed-intensity exercise, the amount of creatine phosphate in the leg was 53 percent greater than it was before creatine ingestion. This was also the first study to actually measure the impact that creatine supplements have on the levels of lactic acid found within the muscle fibers. (The other studies measured blood levels outside of the muscle.) Balsom found that lactic-acid concentrations within muscles dropped by 41 percent. This is an interesting finding, since lactic acid is one of the main causes of muscle fatigue.

The researchers then did the second part of the experiment. They had the volunteers perform a ten-second maximum-intensity workout, and found that creatine supplementation increased the amount of work performed by 5 percent. Despite this greater work effort, muscle lactate levels were 18 percent lower than they were after the men completed their exercise protocol without creatine. There were also increases of 15 percent in total creatine content and 53 percent in creatine phosphate levels. There was a 12 percent rise in the amount of ATP remaining in the muscle tissue as well, which shows that creatine supplements permit quicker resynthesis of valuable ATP.

The Balsom study also showed an overall increase in body mass of 2.4 pounds (1.1 kilograms) after just six days of creatine supplementation. This was a one percent rise in the average body weight of the study participants. The scientists found, however, that there was no improvement in jump performance as a result of creatine ingestion. In this instance, it would appear that the greater strength and increased (heavier) muscle mass that creatine provides balance each other out, so there was no net change in performance.

The Proof Is In The Powder

In a review article published in 1995 in the *International Journal of Sport Nutrition*, Dr. Paul Greenhaff from Queens Medical Centre Department of Physiology in Nottingham, England, confidently states that

research concerned with the effects of creatine ingestion on muscle function and metabolism during exercise in healthy, normal individuals and in disease states is in its infancy, but is sure to progress rapidly. Recent findings indicate that it is important to optimize tissue-creatine uptake in order to maximize performance benefits. Creatine should not be viewed as another gimmick supplement; its ingestion is a means of providing immediate, significant performance improvements to athletes involved in explosive sports. In the long run, creatine may also allow athletes to train with-out fatigue at an intensity higher than that to which they are accustomed. For these reasons alone, creatine supple-mentation could be viewed as a significant development in sport nutrition.

CHAPTER 3

PERSONAL STORIES AND SURVEY OF CREATINE USERS

There is no question that creatine is an effective ergogenic aid. A large number of scientific studies have proven that creatine supplementation increases strength, power, and muscle mass. However, all of these studies were conducted for a period of no more than one month. So, while they are suggestive of the probable long-term benefits that creatine provides, they do not specifically measure how individuals respond to creatine use over the course of several months or years. In order to determine the real-world experiences of users, we conducted a survey of fifty men and women who are currently active in sports. We also interviewed ten of them at length to provide you with a more detailed profile of their personal experiences.

Francis Benfatto

Francis Benfatto was born in Casablanca, Morocco, and moved with his family to France when he was young.

His father was a bodybuilder too, so Francis was surrounded with the sport while he was growing up. He started to lift his father's dumbbells at age 8. Francis also competed as a boxer in his youth, and won a horseback-riding championship.

This professional bodybuilder started working out in a gym at age 15. His intense approach to training and his superior genetics combined to ensure rapid progress at the competitive level. He won the title of Mr. Teenage France at age 17, later dominating the Mr. France contest in 1982. After a strong showing at the 1987 Mr. Universe contest, he turned professional, competing in the Mr. Olympia contest in 1989 and 1990. Since then, Francis has alternated living in France and the United States. He currently calls Venice, California, his home.

Who's Taking Creatine

The athletes who responded to our survey participate in a variety of sports. While most are bodybuilders, several powerlifters and martial artists are also represented. There are track and field athletes, tennis players, and boxers as well. Ninety-two percent of these athletes are men, while only 8 percent are women.

The average age of the men is 34 years, although athletes as young as 19 and as old as 53 contributed to the survey. The typical male athlete is 5 feet 10 inches and 200 pounds after making his gains on creatine. The four women who answered our survey are all in their mid-30s, with an average body weight of 123 pounds.

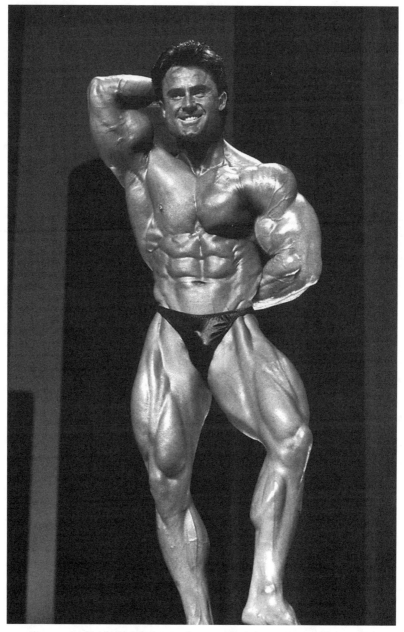

**Francis Benfatto has always had superior shape.
Creatine helped him to add size and chisel his mass
to symmetrical perfection.**

When we interviewed Francis Benfatto, he had only been using creatine for two months. Still, he has found the supplement to be highly effective. Francis has made creatine the central element of his new strategy to stay big and defined without the use of steroids. He feels that creatine is most helpful when he takes it before and after a workout. "Creatine helps me by giving me strength. This lets me do more repetitions as I push myself to exhaustion. I also recover twice as quickly as I did before, so I can hit the weights sooner and maximize my intensity."

Francis also feels that creatine gives him a better "pump," as the muscles become engorged with blood. This sensation inspires him to train even harder. "I get excited when I see my muscles grow. I feel big and very strong, so my training is more rewarding. The added endurance that creatine provides also allows me to get through my entire workout without losing concentration and motivation. I definitely plan to keep on using it." Francis takes 5 grams of creatine before his training session, plus 5 or 10 grams after his workout, depending on whether he is training minor or major body parts that day.

Joe Lazzaro

Joe Lazzaro is another athlete with bodybuilding in the family blood. The middleweight winner of the 1995 Mr. USA contest is the son of Joe Lazzaro, Sr., who won the Mr. North America contest in the early 1960s. Joe is a life-long sports enthusiast. He has been playing hockey since he was 6 years old, and played collegiate hockey while earning his bachelor of science degree from the

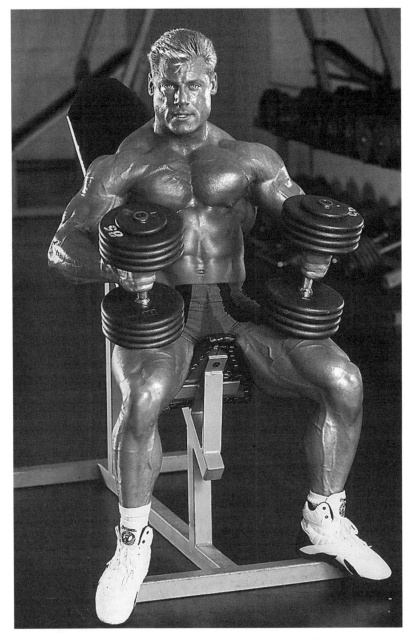

Joe Lazzaro gained seven pounds of muscle during a year of creatine use, compared to the one- or two-pound annual gains he had achieved previously.

University of Buffalo. When he decided not to become a professional hockey player, he turned his considerable athletic talents to bodybuilding.

Joe started training with weights ten years ago. The very next year he won the Teenage Mr. Buffalo contest. In rapid succession, he then won the overall titles of Mr. Buffalo and Mr. New York State, and the middleweight title at the Jr. USA. He still lives in Buffalo, where he teaches physics and biology in high school. Joe is currently finishing up his master's degree in science education.

Creatine has helped Joe make dramatic improvements. In the past year he has gained seven pounds of solid muscle, compared to the one- or two-pound annual gains he had achieved previously. He started taking creatine right after his USA win, and decided to skip the loading phase. "I'm very sensitive to supplements, so I wanted to ease into creatine use. Despite the low-calorie diet I stayed on after the USA contest to remain in top shape for guest-posing appearances, I gained two to three pounds of lean mass in the first week, and saw exciting strength gains by the second week. I also found it reduced my joint inflammation."

Joe feels there is value in cycling creatine use. His cycles last eight to ten weeks, and he has gone through four cycles so far. He thinks that the body can get accustomed to creatine supplementation, so he feels it makes sense to take time off every once in a while. Joe also thinks that creatine can produce a small amount of subcutaneous water retention. While this amount of water would not normally be a problem, in today's super-competitive bodybuilding contests it can make the difference between winning and placing. As a result, Joe stops taking creatine three weeks before a show. His usual dosage is 10 to 15 grams per day.

Marla Duncan

When she was in high school, Marla Duncan was faced with two options. She could either take jazzercise or weightlifting for her required PE class. The weights won, and since then, bodybuilding has been an integral part of Marla's life. She quickly became addicted to how good she felt and how people reacted to her ever-improving physique. Although she has tried her hand at virtually every sport, she chose bodybuilding as the outlet for her competitive spirit. She entered her first fitness show in 1989, and soon won the coveted Ms. Fitness USA title. She also works as a model and writer, and stars in a cable TV show called *Training and Nutrition 2000*.

In the year since Marla began taking creatine, she has added ten pounds of muscle to her 125 pound frame. "Creatine made a marked, visible difference for me," she says. "I'm a vegetarian, so I didn't have as much creatine in my muscles when I started supplementing. The changes were quick and very noticeable." Marla added an inch to her calves in nine months, helping her overcome what she considered a flaw in her physique. Creatine also allowed her to drop her body fat level by 3 percent, even though her cardiovascular exercise routine was unchanged and her diet was a bit "looser" than it used to be. She has noticed improvements in her workout recovery as well.

Marla has seen dramatic progress in her definition and vascularity while using the supplement. Yet these gains appear to be temporary. In fact, when she cycled off creatine after an eight-week period, her husband noticed that she "went flat" almost immediately. Still,

---

Gains From Creatine Use

Both men and women report dramatic gains from creatine supplementation. The average man gained eight pounds of body weight, which is a 4 percent increase in his total mass. Male athletes reported weight gains ranging from zero to twenty pounds. Those with the greatest initial muscle mass noted the largest gains in total size. Many men also indicated that their body fat level dropped simultaneously with the increases in body weight. This drop in body fat averaged 2.5 percent. Since total body weight is the sum of lean mass plus body fat, their total gains in lean mass were actually higher than the gains in body weight. The estimated increase in lean mass was thirteen pounds, which represents a 7.5 percent rise in total lean mass. Nearly all of these gains occurred during the first six months of creatine use.

Women made even greater improvements from a percentage standpoint. Their average gain in total body weight was 5 percent (1 percent more than the men). They also reported a greater drop in body fat (3 percent), so their increase in total lean mass was a whopping 9 percent! Because of their smaller frames, however, women had fewer pounds of muscle gain. The average increase in total body weight was six pounds, while the corresponding rise in lean mass was ten pounds.

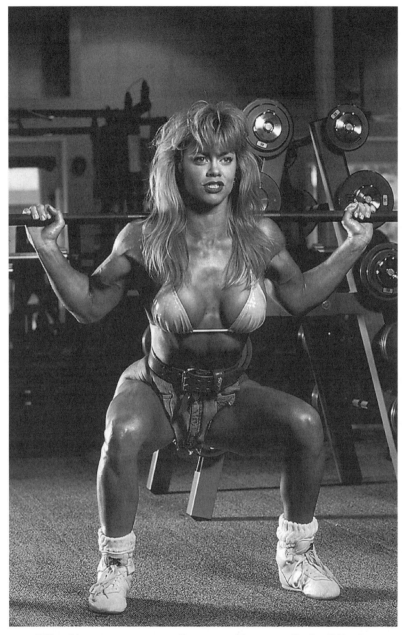

The improvements that creatine made in Marla Duncan's physique were even quicker and more visible because she is a vegetarian.

Marla feels that the benefits of creatine use are great. "If you're not taking creatine, you're not giving your work-

Loading Strategies

Most users do a loading phase when they start taking creatine. This fills up their muscles with the nutrient and allows them to see the benefits of creatine use relatively quickly. Our survey revealed, however, that some 15 percent choose not to load. The reasons for this vary from a desire to start experimenting with a light dose and see what the effects are, to a lack of awareness about the advantages of a loading phase.

Men and women have the same average loading dosage: 20 grams per day. Men have a wider range in their loading strategies, with some taking a little as 10 grams and others loading with as much as 40 grams per day. Women tend to stay closer to the average, with a range of 10 to 30 grams. This may be due to an understanding among women that the amount of creatine needed for loading is directly related to muscle mass.

The average loading phase for men lasts seven days, although two men loaded for only three days and another loaded for forty-two days. Most men divide their daily dosage into three or four servings, which results in an average serving of 5 to 7 grams. The typical loading strategy for women is similar to that of men. Women usually load for six days and divide their 20-gram loading phase into three servings per day.

out the best you can give it," she says. Marla does a one-week loading phase of 30 grams per day, and then takes 5 grams a day for her maintenance dose.

Jeff Ward

Jeff is a 24-year-old medical student. He has trained for many years and packs a solid 223 pounds on his 5-foot 9-inch frame. Jeff has used creatine on and off for the last four years with remarkably positive results. He experimented with various levels of creatine use, and found that he needs to take more creatine than is usually recommended in order to make the greatest gains.

His first creatine cycle lasted four weeks. Jeff took 25 grams for five days as a loading dose. His maintenance dosage was 10 grams on non-workout days and 15 grams on workout days. During this cycle he went from 192 to 197 pounds, and he noticed good strength gains, especially during the fourth week. Unfortunately, the four-week cycle was too short to permit the assembly of permanent structural proteins in the muscle cells, so most of the initial "volumizing" gains were due to intra-cellular water. As a result, he lost four of the five pounds he gained on his first cycle.

Jeff's next three cycles lasted eight to ten weeks each. He upped his loading dose to 40 grams a day, which he divided into five 8-gram servings. His loading phase lasted seven days, two days more than before. Jeff also increased his maintenance dose to 18 grams on non-workout days and 24 grams on the days he trained. He divided this dose into three to four 6-gram servings,

which he always took on an empty stomach. Jeff is metic-
ulous about his creatine supplementation. "I dissolve my
creatine in three ounces of grape juice per gram of creatine, and always take a vanadyl sulfate tablet along with
it. Both of these things, I feel, greatly increase the effects
of creatine. I also spread my creatine dosage throughout
the day, with one serving right after waking up, another
immediately after my workout (yes, I bring it to the
gym!), and one or two more servings in between meals."

Maintenance Strategies

Our average creatine user has been taking the supplement for six months. The time that individuals
have been on creatine, however, ranges from two
weeks to four years. After the loading phase, most
men continue on a maintenance dosage of 10
grams, which is usually divided into two servings.
The actual individual dose is variable, ranging
from 1 to 24 grams per day.

Although the vast majority of men take the same
amount of creatine every day, 12 percent vary their
dosage depending on their workout schedule. One
surveyed athlete takes creatine only on the days he
works out, while the others reduce their maintenance dose on the days they don't train.

Women usually maintain their creatine supplementation with a daily dose of either 5 or 10 grams.
This is taken in one or two servings. No women in
the survey indicated that they modify their creatine consumption on off-days.

During Jeff's last cycle, he went from 215 to 223 pounds while losing body fat, so he had an even greater increase in lean mass. He is still 223 pounds, so he didn't lose an ounce of his gains during his last off-cycle. Meanwhile, he is stronger than ever. He is now benching 365 pounds for four repetitions, doing narrow-grip pulldowns with 400 pounds for six reps, and blasting out ten reps on the leg press with 1,415 pounds piled on. To say that he is excited with his gains would be a gross understatement!

Gold's Powerlifting Team

They are a fixture at Gold's Gym, Venice. Four nights each week, and on Saturday mornings, seven very intense powerlifters meet to train under the direction of nationally ranked powerlifter and coach Kurt Elder. In a gym that has more than its share of big athletes, this team sets the standard for heavy lifting. Eyes inevitably turn as these lifters pile on the plates and practice for their bench press, deadlift, and squatting events. Now, however, you can hear the clanging of even more plates than usual. The Gold's powerlifting team has discovered creatine.

Coach Kurt Elder has been powerlifting for over eight years, acquiring an impressive list of first-place awards from 1988 to 1994. He also has a claim to fame as the model for the internationally recognized Gold's Gym logo. When he decided to retire from competition due to a shoulder injury, he started working with some members of the present team. Over time, the group developed into the current seven members.

Kurt says that three people in the group are using creatine at this time. All of them made impressive gains in strength and power, with noticeable improvements with-

The Many Benefits Of Creatine Use

Our survey respondents listed a wide range of benefits from the use of creatine. The most common were greater muscle mass, increased strength, quicker recovery, reduced body fat, and more energy. Since the survey form did not include a checklist of possible benefits, everyone had to write in the gains they experienced. Some survey responses were more comprehensive than others. As a result, the actual types of benefits and the percentage of athletes who felt them may be greater than indicated below.

Men were most impressed with the size they gained on creatine. Eighty-two percent said they increased their lean muscle mass while using the supplement. Another 77 percent mentioned that they had more strength, while 39 percent claimed quicker recovery and/or improved endurance. About a third (34 percent) of the respondents also noted that creatine reduced their body fat level and increased their definition or vascularity. An additional 26 percent listed greater energy as a benefit from creatine use. Other benefits listed include more power and work output, less fatigue, more stamina, greater agility and explosiveness, and an increased "pump."

All of the women responding to the survey commented on the increased strength they got from creatine. Seventy-five percent also noted improvements in definition or vascularity, along with greater lean muscle mass. Additional benefits include improved recovery from workouts and less muscle soreness.

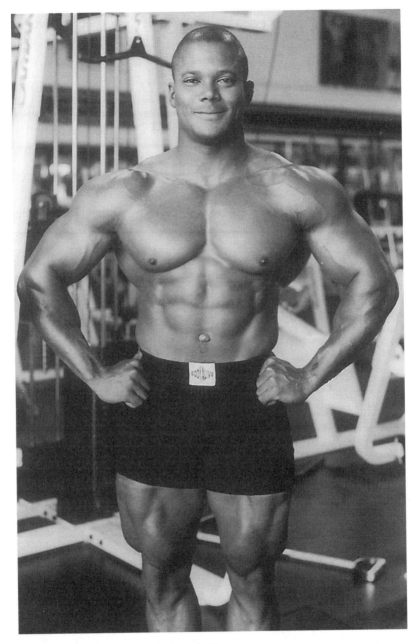

Powerlifting coach Kurt Elder says his lifters make impressive gains in strength and power after only two weeks of creatine supplementation.

in two weeks. We were able to interview two of these creatine users. We also talked with one of the lifters who has stayed away from creatine supplementation for now.

Mike Laney studies physiology at UCLA. He joined the powerlifting team a year ago after he met Kurt at a meet. Mike made major progress in his lifts during the first six months, but then his gains stalled out. Sometimes he would even "die" in the middle of a set. While he had heard about creatine before, he wasn't convinced that the claims for it were true. Still, he decided to take the plunge, and now he's glad he did. Mike reports exciting gains in strength. His bench press rose from 342 to 370 pounds and his squat increased from 595 to 633 pounds, while his deadlift jumped from 640 to 688 pounds. He's also added twenty pounds to his body weight, topping the 200-pound mark for the first time in his life. Mike also says he has more endurance with creatine, so he can push harder on every set. He plans to keep using it for a long time.

Kristine Emry is the only woman currently on the team. She has been a competitive lifter for two years, and has picked up a closet-full of trophies for her efforts. Kristine has used creatine for only six weeks so far, but she already feels much stronger. Her deadlift has risen from 235 to 275 pounds and her squat has jumped from 225 to 265 pounds—more than twice her 112-pound body weight. Kristine has also seen her body fat level drop by 4 percent, while her lean mass has increased by eight pounds. All in all, the therapist for neglected or abused youth at the Long Beach Boys Town is very happy with her results. Kristine can hardly wait for her next competition!

John Arenberg is not your typical rocket scientist. While this Ph.D. in engineering does work with the TRW Space Program, he packs incredible strength into his 5-foot frame. John won the 123 pound class at the U.S. Powerlifting Federation's Senior Nationals in 1995, and took eighth at the USPF World Championships that same year. John has worked with Kurt for over five years, and they frequently brainstorm on kinesiology and nutrition. John has also done research on creatine, and for now has decided to avoid creatine use. The reason: he knows it works! John is at the top of his weight class, and he recognizes that the strength and mass gains which creatine provides will push him into the next weight group. This could mean taking time off from competition until he builds up to the next weight limit, something he is presently unwilling to do.

Marius Dinu

Marius has been involved in the martial arts since he was thirteen years old. His teacher, Jerry Smith, was taught by the legendary Bruce Lee, and much of Bruce's knowledge and expertise have been passed on to Marius. He has achieved the master's level in six of the martial arts, including karate, tae kwon do, hapkido, aikido, Chinese kenpo, and Okinawan shorin ryu. He is currently working on becoming a grand master. Marius has taught the martial arts since 1988, and loves to show others the intricate nuances of these detailed art forms. He also finds it a great way to stay in shape.

Marius has used creatine on and off for a year and a half. During this period he gained eight pounds of solid muscle, with most of the gain occurring in the first six months. He finds that the power and strength gains pro-

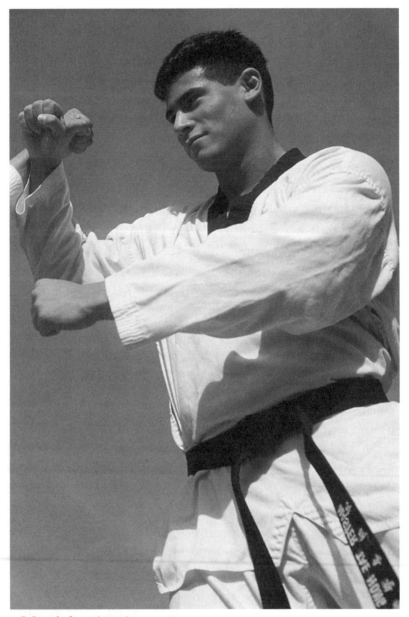

**Martial artists have discovered that creatine boosts
the explosiveness of their actions, allowing them
to perform quicker combinations of punches
and kicking movements.**

Side Effects

While there are no negative complications reported in the medical literature on creatine, the people responding to our survey indicate that creatine can sometimes produce minor side effects if not used appropriately. None of the survey respondents reported any toxicity or side effect serious enough to make them discontinue their use of the supplement. However, 38 percent of the men and 25 percent of the women mentioned some temporary side effect connected with their creatine use.

The most common complaint among men was mild diarrhea. Seventeen percent of the men said they experienced loose stools during the loading phase, particularly when the serving size was greater than 10 grams. Taking creatine on an empty stomach also increases the chances of getting diarrhea, according to some users. This problem appears to go away when the serving size is reduced to 5 grams.

Eight percent of the men surveyed said they had occasional gas or flatulence, while 6 percent complained of an upset stomach or stomach cramps, particularly during the loading phase. All of these conditions responded to changes in the serving size or total dosage level.

The remaining 7 percent of the men noted a variety of additional side effects, many of which could have been the result of other dietary or lifestyle practices. They could also be due to the other ingredients which are sometimes included in creatine-based products. Increased urination, headaches or reduced appetite were mentioned by two users each during the period they were supplementing with creatine. Nervousness, irritability, bloating, sleepiness, a drop in sex drive, and skin blotching were each indicated by one man. While there is no evidence to connect creatine with any of these conditions, nor even a theory as to why creatine might be responsible, we are presenting you with this information to keep this book totally objective.

Women have not reported any ongoing problems with creatine use. Only one woman said she got nauseated when she took creatine on an empty stomach. The problem went away when she consumed the supplement with a meal.

vided by creatine are the most helpful benefits for the martial arts. The enhanced energy he gets from the supplement also allows him to increase his work output and boosts the explosiveness of his actions. This enables him to perform quicker combinations of punches and kicking movements. Creatine increases his agility as well.

North Hollywood Police Station

Competitive athletes are not the only people who have discovered the benefits of creatine. At the North Hollywood Station of the Los Angeles Police Department, five police officers have experimented with the supplement for periods ranging from six to eight months. They have found that the increased strength and endurance which creatine provides helps them perform their duties better. They can now run quicker and apprehend criminals with greater ease, allowing them to preserve the peace more effectively. We were able to interview two of the officers for this book.

Nick Zingo is a police lieutenant. He was the first person at the station to try creatine. Nick has been bodybuilding for four years now, and continues to run four to five miles after each workout. He experienced immediate gains in strength and performance after taking the supplement. "With creatine, I'm raring to go to the gym. I've also found that it boosts my endurance and increases the speed of my runs." The 21-year veteran of the police force also gained five pounds of muscle mass, even though his running makes it hard for him to put on size. Nick is definitely sold on creatine. "In fact, I wouldn't be without it," he says.

Officer John Smith works out with Nick at the Powerhouse Gym in nearby Chatsworth. After Nick got such positive results from creatine, John decided to try it for himself. He discovered that creatine adds a lot more physical power and strength to his workouts. He also feels that he recovers from the stresses of training more quickly than before. This has helped him in his line of work. The explosive energy he gets from creatine allows him to run faster, so he can catch more criminals in the act. John can also arrive at the scene sooner, sometimes ending a fight before it starts.

With experiences such as these, creatine may well become standard issue for public safety officers in the future. Just imagine: as they cross the stage to get their diplomas and badges, graduates of police academies could even be handed a kilo of creatine!

CHAPTER 4

HOW MUCH TO TAKE
AND WHEN

O
ne of the most important decisions for a creatine
user is determining the right amount of creatine
to take. Your dosage and frequency of use need
to be appropriate to achieve the benefits you seek, yet
should not be so high as to overload your body's ability
to assimilate this nutrient. Clearly, there is no advantage
to consuming so much creatine that part of your dose
winds up flushing out of your plumbing. Although no
studies are available to indicate this, it is theoretically
possible that excessive creatine, in the long run, could
potentially stress your organs of metabolism and elimination, such as the liver and kidneys. More is not necessarily better. This chapter will discuss the proper dosages
of creatine for athletes, the general public, seniors, and
teenagers.

There are two ways you can ingest creatine: through
certain foods and as a supplement.

Foods That Contain Creatine

One way to get part of the creatine you need is to consume the skeletal muscle of animals. Just as human muscle contains creatine, so does the muscle of most mammals and fish. As you can see in Table 1, the amount of creatine in most meats and fish is relatively constant, staying within a narrow range of 4 to 5 grams per kilogram (2.2 pounds). Cod has a lower amount because of its high water content. While it seems logical that chicken and turkey also contain creatine, the precise quantity of this nutrient in these meats has not yet been determined.

Table 1
Foods Containing Creatine

Food	Creatine Content (g/kg)
Meat and Fish	
Beef	4.5
Chicken	NA
Cod	3.0
Herring	6.5
Pork	5.0
Salmon	4.5
Tuna	4.0
Turkey	NA
Other Sources	
Cranberries	0.02
Milk	0.1

NA = Not Available

While you can get some of the creatine you need from these protein sources, you shouldn't dramatically increase your meat and fish consumption in order to pump your muscles full of this nutrient. Remember that meats and fish contain a lot more than creatine. All animal flesh contains relatively high amounts of cholesterol, which has been associated with hardening of the arteries (atherosclerosis). Also, most meats, especially beef and pork, contain high quantities of saturated fats. For example, 2.2 pounds (one kilogram) of raw round steak contains only 4 grams of creatine, but has 119 grams of fat. Porterhouse steak has a bit less creatine, but 325 grams of fat per kilo! You won't live to see your 90s if you ingest the amount of meat you would need to improve your strength and power. You'll simply clog your arteries. Moreover, this fat content can dramatically increase the total number of calories you consume each day. Unless your exercise intensity and volume increase at the same rate, you will wind up gaining unwanted pounds of body fat. A far better solution is to take the non-fat, no-cholesterol supplement known as creatine monohydrate.

The Loading Phase

The concept of a loading phase came from scientific studies done in the early 1990s. A 1992 study by Harris found that a low dose of creatine monohydrate (1 gram) produced only modest increases in the blood level of creatine and no appreciable increase in muscle. On the other hand, 5 grams given four to six times per day resulted in a sustained rise in blood levels and a significant accumulation of creatine in muscle fibers. It was therefore felt that higher creatine levels in muscle could only be achieved if there was a consistent elevation in the amount of creatine in the blood stream over a prolonged period of time.

The question then became how long this loading period had to be. It turns out not to be that long at all. Harris gave his study subjects 30 grams of creatine per day, which by today's standards is a very high dose, even for the loading phase. Study participants weighed around 175 pounds (80 kilograms) and engaged in only light exercise during the course of the study. Harris found that the muscles could absorb only so much creatine. After the maximum level had been reached, the excess amount was converted into a waste product called creatinine and excreted in the urine. Harris discovered that on the first day of supplementation, 40 percent of the administered dose was excreted. This amount rose to 61 percent on the second day and 68 percent on the third day. So by day three, two-thirds of the creatine consumed was wasted!

An unpublished study referred to by Dr. Balsom in his review article shows the effectiveness of the loading and maintenance concept. In this study, participants received 0.3 grams of creatine per kilogram of bodyweight every day for six days. (For a 70-kilogram person, this would be 21 grams per day.) That dose produced a significant increase in total creatine levels in skeletal muscle. Creatinine excretion was not measured. After this loading phase, the amount of creatine was reduced to 0.03 grams per day per kilogram, which is roughly equal to 2 grams per day for a 70-kilogram person. On this low dose, muscle creatine levels were maintained at the high level originally brought about by the loading phase. Unfortunately, the research did not reveal how much the participants exercised, if at all. Nevertheless, this study indicated that high loading dosages of creatine do not need to be continued over a long period of time.

If you keep taking high doses of creatine after your muscles have been loaded, you're basically unloading; that is, unloading your cash. Your money is being flushed down the toilet. As mentioned earlier, it's also possible that excessive doses of creatine could place stress on some of your organs, such as your liver and kidneys. Your body would have to work harder to get rid of all that excess creatine, and that's not healthy.

Although a loading phase can provide you with quicker and more noticeable gains within days of use, it is not necessary if you are willing to be patient. A 1996 study by Hultman showed that in people who did not exercise, a dosage of 3 grams per day for a month was as effective at raising tissue levels of creatine as a 20 gram, six-day loading phase followed by 2 grams per day for the rest of the month.

The Maintenance Phase

The maintenance phase is the period of time after your loading phase. Once you have filled your muscles with creatine to their maximum capacity, you only need to consume enough creatine to keep your storage bins full at all times. It's similar to topping off the tank of your car's gasoline supply. That way you can gain all of the benefits of creatine supplementation without placing undue stress on your kidneys. However, as we men-

Table 2
Loading and Maintenance Dosages
for Athletes (in grams)

Loading Dosages

Body Weight	Workout Level		
	1	2	3
Up to 175 lb. (up to 80 kg)	12	14	16
176 – 225 lb. (81 – 100 kg)	14	16	18
Over 225 lb. (over 100 kg)	16	18	20

Maintenance Dosages

Body Weight	Workout Level		
	1	2	3
Up to 175 lb. (up to 80 kg)	4	5	6
176 – 225 lb. (81 – 100 kg)	6	7	8
Over 225 lb. (over 100 kg)	8	9	10

Workout Levels

Level 1: One hour of training, two to three times per week, at a low level of intensity.

Level 2: Two hours of training, three to four times per week, at a medium level of intensity.

Level 3: Three hours of training, five to six times per week, at a high level of intensity.

---

tioned above, the loading phase is optional. If you want to begin slowly, you can skip the loading phase and begin with the maintenance dose.

Maintenance dosages are related to your exercise level, age, bodyweight, and whether you want to look like Mr. Universe or just toned. All these factors influence the amount of creatine you need. The higher your workout level, the more creatine you will metabolize during your physical activity. Also, the more muscle you have, the more storage capacity you have to keep full. Servings should be no more than 5 grams, since larger doses can cause diarrhea. You should also drink 8 ounces of water with each dose.

Later in the chapter, we'll discuss the appropriate dosages for several groups of users, including the general public, seniors, and teenagers.

Recommendations for Athletes

At the present time, we recommend a high-dose loading phase only for athletes eager to bulk up quickly. As you can see from Table 2, the total daily dosage ranges from

12 to 20 grams, depending on your body weight and exercise intensity. This dosage should be divided into two to four servings. Servings should generally not be greater than 5 grams since larger doses, in some instances, can produce nausea, weakness, dizziness, and diarrhea. You should also drink 8 ounces of water with each dose. The loading phase should last from five to seven days if you are a meat-eater, and seven to ten days if you are vegetarian. (Vegetarians have lower initial levels of creatine stored in muscles.)

During the loading phase, you should increase your workout intensity only gradually. While the increase in muscle mass and strength can give athletes the feeling that they can rapidly raise the amount of weight they lift or the number of repetitions they do, this boost in exercise intensity could potentially place undue stress on tendons and ligaments that have not had time to adapt to the increase in muscular strength. We know one athlete who temporarily strained his right elbow when he added weight to his barbells too quickly. The increase in muscle mass made him overconfident and unreasonably enthusiastic.

Table 2 also includes recommendations for maintenance dosages. Since the consequences of continuous daily use for months or years currently are not known, we recommend that you refrain from creatine use for one or two weeks a few times per year. It's better to be on the cautious side until more research is published on the long-term use of creatine.

The recommendations in Table 2 are based on two major factors. First, the total amount of creatine storage capacity in your body is directly related to your muscle mass. Ninety-five percent of the body's creatine is found in skeletal muscles. There is no creatine in bones or body fat, and only small amounts in the heart, brain, and testes. Also, while there are some variations in the creatine content of individual muscles, every kilogram of muscle (2.2 pounds) has, on average, around 4 grams of creatine in it. As a result, the more muscle you have, the greater the quantity of storage space available. This increases the amount of creatine you need to load proportionally.

Second, the amount of creatine you need depends on your exercise program. Even a sedentary 155-pound (70-kilogram) person uses up 2 grams of creatine each day. Rates of creatine metabolism for active individuals are much higher. Consequently, you will be "burning" part of your creatine dosage every day. This means that not all of your loading and maintenance doses goes into your muscles' storage bins. Part of it gets used up for fuel during your workouts. The amount consumed, of course, depends on the workout level of your exercise routine, which is a combination of its length, intensity, and frequency. While creatine will help you gain muscle mass, taking too much, too soon can definitely set you back, particularly if you wind up getting diarrhea from the overdose. (Try putting on weight while you spend half the day in the bathroom!)

Recommendations for the General Public

You don't have to be a competitive athlete to benefit from creatine. We feel that almost everyone who wants a better-looking body can take advantage of creatine's ability to tone muscles. By tailoring the amount of creatine you take to your specific needs, you can determine how much muscle mass and strength you will gain.

Unless you need to see immediate results, we recommend you skip the loading phase. This way, you will minimize the potential side effects of nausea or diarrhea that can occur from the high doses of creatine used for loading. The following are some general recommendations. These are not set in stone, and you may wish to take less or more, depending on your particular desires and amount of physical activity.

1) Skip the loading phase.
2) Use 3 to 6 grams every other day, as a
   maintenance dose.
3) Take one week off per month.
4) Take one complete month off, two or three times
   per year.

We recommend that you take these breaks because we wish to be cautious in our recommendations. Until thorough, long-term studies of continuous creatine use are completed, it is best to use creatine conservatively.

A Note to Seniors

We believe that a great, untapped potential for creatine has been overlooked—its use in middle-aged and older individuals.

One of the frustrations of aging is that our muscles gradually start to shrink. It becomes increasingly difficult to regain the bulk we once had. Putting in a lot of hours at the gym, going on long walks or runs, or playing many sets of tennis don't seem to give the rewards they once did. The muscles just don't respond the way they used to.

Older individuals with decreased muscle mass can significantly benefit from creatine supplementation. Since creatine boosts strength and protein synthesis and aids in the storage of water in muscle cells, it should help to reduce the muscle wasting that can occur with disease and the aging process. Being more muscular can also lead to an improved sense of self-esteem and well-being. Older individuals can look and feel years younger. Stronger muscles may also lead to fewer falls and bone fractures. Some users who "bulk up" report feeling more sexually attractive.

The studies that used high doses of creatine, such as 20 grams per day, have been done with young, healthy volunteers. Until more research is done with seniors, we recommend that older individuals use lower dosages. The dosages for seniors are slightly lower than those for the general public. If you have a chronic medical condition or are on medication, consult a physician before using creatine. You should:

1) Skip the loading phase.
2) Use 3 to 4 grams every other day, as a
   maintenance dose.
3) Take one week off per month.
4) Take one complete month off, two or three times
   per year.

Creatine and Teenagers

Since the first few printings of this book, we have had many calls and inquiries from high school and college coaches who want to know whether creatine is appropriate for teenagers. We have struggled to find a suitable response to this question. On one hand, we don't want teenagers to rely on supplements for their athletic performance. At the same time, if other teen athletes were using creatine, non-users would be at a competitive disadvantage. And any attempt to enforce a ban on creatine use for teenagers would not work, because the supplement is easily available over the counter. Moreover, some high school athletes have relied on synthetic anabolic steroids as a way to increase muscle mass, and creatine is a much safer way to increase muscle size and strength.

Having weighed both sides of the issue, we feel that teens should use only small amounts of creatine (in the 3 to 5 gram daily range) for a limited period of time. For instance, a high school athlete could use creatine for a couple of months during the football season and then avoid using the supplement until the next season. This moderate approach may be satisfactory to the athlete, while helping to resolve the concerns of coaches and the teenager's family.

The Best Way to Take Creatine

Creatine monohydrate is a white powder that looks like table sugar. It is odorless and virtually tasteless. While creatine should be consumed with at least 4 to 8 ounces of liquid, some liquids are better than others. This is because the shuttle system used to transport creatine into the muscle fibers involves insulin, so you want to mix your creatine with a liquid that will cause a temporary increase, or spike, in the insulin level of your blood. This can dramatically increase the amount of creatine that gets transported into your muscle cells, while reducing the amount that is excreted. Almost all the research studies to date have used glucose as a sugar source. A study by Green found that creatine concentrations in muscle rose an additional 60 percent on average when the study participants added nearly 100 grams of simple sugars to the 5 grams of creatine they consumed. One hundred grams is quite a load of sugar, and it may not be healthy to consume this amount on a regular basis. Anecdotal evidence suggests that smaller amounts of carbohydrates are also effective.

Fruit and vegetable juices are good options. Juices contain large amounts of fructose and other simple sugars. These are assimilated relatively quickly, so they are perfectly acceptable as a creatine vehicle. Furthermore, fruit and vegetable juices contain significant amounts of vitamins, minerals, carotenoids, and flavonoids. We mix our creatine in 3 to 4 ounces of juice along with a few ounces of water. Be aware that excessive doses of creatine can cause loose stools. Therefore, the one drink we don't recommend is prune juice, for obvious reasons. You could also mix your creatine with a combination protein/carbohydrate drink, although the protein content of the drink may slow the assimilation of the creatine, compared to glucose alone. Some individuals even take creatine with meals. Although the fat and protein in a meal may reduce the insulin spike achieved, anecdotal evidence suggests that the creatine is still absorbed by the muscle cells, as long as the meal contains sufficient carbohydrates. Mixing creatine with food also minimizes any gastrointestinal discomfort and may be a preferred option for people with sensitive stomachs.

People have sometimes been told to avoid the use of citrus juices, such as orange juice, with creatine. The reason given is that the acidity in these juices boosts the production of creatinine, which is the waste product of creatine metabolism. However, creatinine is formed in the muscles, not in a glass. Moreover, the citric acid in orange and grapefruit juices is insignificant compared to the concentrated hydrochloric acid found in the stomach. If creatine can make it through the stomach and into the body, a little bit of o.j. won't hurt. On the other hand, one study by Vandenberghe shows that the benefits of creatine are counteracted when it is consumed with large amounts of caffeine (the equivalent of 10 cups of coffee). The study found that while caffeine did not reduce the increase in creatine-phosphate levels within the muscle fibers, dynamic torque production in caffeine/creatine' users was 10 to 20 percent lower than in test subjects who took creatine alone. In fact, torque production for the caffeine/creatine users was no different than the placebo group. Based on this research, you should definitely stay away from high-potency caffeine pills. Mixing creatine in caffeinated drinks, at least according to this study, may also reduce or even neutralize performance-enhancing effects of this nutrient in the short term. It's better to take your creatine with a glucose- or fructose-based drink that will stimulate your insulin response and facilitate the uptake of creatine into the muscle fibers.

The Best Time to Take Creatine

Creatine remains in the blood stream for a period of one to two hours. This is the window of opportunity that muscles have to draw creatine from the surrounding blood vessels and store it in their cells. If these cells are full of creatine, and the brain, heart, and testes have all of the creatine they need, the excess eventually will be processed into creatinine and excreted.

Therefore, timing is important. You want to make sure that the maximum amount of creatine is absorbed by your muscles and not wasted. The ideal times to take creatine are before and after your workouts. Taking it before exercise allows the nutrient to circulate in the blood during your routine, so your muscles can quickly replenish the creatine metabolized during exercise. Consuming it after your workout improves recovery and helps to stimulate additional protein uptake and synthesis in the critical hour after the end of exercise. If you are dividing your daily maintenance dose into only two parts, take at least one of them before or after your workout. If you are loading, include these two times along with others spread throughout the day. This will give your muscles several windows of opportunity over a 24-hour period.

While these suggestions will help you to maximize the gains you get from creatine, it's important to keep things in perspective. Creatine is not a nutrient that flushes out of your system in a short time. Unlike water-soluble vitamins, which cannot be stored by the body, creatine accumulates in your muscle cells. This means that the whole issue of timing is not as critical as it is for other nutrients. You're not dealing with an all-or-nothing situation where a matter of hours can make the difference between progress and stagnation. So don't panic if you forget to take a dose with your workout, or even if you skip a day. We promise that you won't shrink. As long as you make regular efforts to keep your creatine stores full, you will achieve the gains reported in the scientific literature.

Cycling

Cycling is a technique frequently employed by persons who use anabolic steroids. A cycle is a length of time divided into on- and off-periods. The purpose of steroid cycling is twofold. First, since steroids put stress on the liver and other organs, the off-cycle allows the athlete's body to recuperate from any damage. Second, since steroid use turns off the body's own testosterone production, the off-cycle allows the testes to temporarily "bounce back."

Because of the common practice of steroid cycling, athletes have sometimes extended its use to creatine. But creatine is not a synthetic hormone and does not impact the body in the same way that steroids do. Creatine is a naturally occurring nutrient that provides additional fuel reserves for your body, allowing it to perform at its best. It is not a foreign substance that the body must process.

Having said this, we still feel that it is wise to take breaks from creatine use. We suggest this because we don't know the long-term effects of daily creatine use over many years. Although there has been no mention in the medical literature of a person's endogenous creatine production shutting off permanently as a result of creatine supplementation, it would be best to take occasional breaks in order to allow the body to make its own creatine. You could cycle creatine on an every-other-day, every-other-week regimen, or follow the recommendations we have outlined in the above sections. Since creatine is trapped within the muscle fibers for an extended period of time, such a routine should not produce any major creatine loss within your muscle tissues, and you should quickly regain most, if not all, of your muscle mass shortly after you start taking creatine again.

Stacking

Stacking refers to the simultaneous administration of two or more different ergogenic aids. Athletes have combined creatine with virtually every supplement on the market, ranging from simple protein powders to vanadyl, chromium, androstenedione, pregnenolone, DHEA (dehydroepiandrosterone) and HMB (hydroxymethylbutyrate). Unfortunately, there has been no published research on this subject to date. However, anecdotal reports and our survey results do not reveal any substances that should definitely be avoided while using creatine. Given the benign nature of creatine and its easy elimination from the body, this is not surprising.

Some athletes have reported that vanadyl sulfate helps them get greater results from creatine. This is probably because vanadyl sulfate has an insulin-like effect, helping to increase amino-acid and glucose entry into the muscles. Since insulin is also involved in the mechanism for creatine uptake, it seems logical that taking a vanadyl supplement along with your creatine would increase the amount of creatine absorbed into the muscle cells. However, there is no research that actually proves this. Try some vanadyl with your creatine if you like, but be sure to stay with the recommended dosages on the bottle. Vanadium is a metal, and cannot be easily excreted from the body. Theoretically, it could build up to toxic levels, so more is not necessarily better.

We have come across anecdotal reports that the combination of creatine with natural hormones and nutrients can produce better results. No scientific studies have been published regarding these combinations. Hormone supplements that could potentially help include androstenedione and DHEA. We do not recommend the regular use of these hormones. They could have androgenic effects leading to pimples, irritability, aggressiveness, and facial hair growth in women. High doses could potentially accelerate hair loss and even stimulate prostate growth in older men. It's likely that older individuals would be more likely to benefit from these hormones since they are more likely to be deficient in them. Younger people generally have adequate amounts of these hormones circulating in their systems. If you are planning to use androstenedione or DHEA, use them only on the days that you work out.

Another combination that has been anecdotally reported as beneficial is creatine with the amino acid glutamine. You may give this combination a try to see if it works for you. Also, tribulus is an herb touted as a muscle enhancer. It is sometimes combined with androstenedione in capsules. We are not aware of any studies evaluating this herb as a muscle builder.

What Happens If I Stop Using Creatine?

You shrink back to a 95-pound weakling and people will throw sand in your face. Just kidding.

After it is absorbed and incorporated within the muscle cells, creatine stays there for days and even weeks. Due to a unique entry process, once creatine enters the muscle fiber, it remains trapped there for a relatively long time. Two studies have shown that creatine levels decline slowly over the course of several weeks when there is no additional supplementation. As time goes on, the muscles gradually lose their additional creatine stores, and some of the results obtained from the supplement disappear. Unfortunately, there has been no extensive research done in this area, so at this point, estimates of loss are pure conjecture. It may well be that part of the muscle mass and strength gained from creatine will continue after supplementation ends. Presently, we don't know for sure.

Caution

Creatine supplements have been found to be remarkably safe. After all, creatine is found in our foods and we consume about a gram per day, on average. However, we don't know for certain what might happen in the long run if people take high dosages continuously for many months or years. Would there be undue stress placed on the liver or kidneys? Would high blood levels of creatine cause some harm that we don't know of yet? Is it possible that the body's internal creatine-production system will shut off permanently if not allowed to exercise its function every once in a while? We don't have the full answers to these questions yet.

Consequently, if you have any medical problems, we recommend that you consult a physician before supplementing with creatine. This is especially important if you have kidney or liver disorders. The kidneys are the main organs responsible for eliminating creatinine, the breakdown product of creatine. Therefore, if you have kidney disease, and you take a high load of creatine, your blood creatinine levels could rise to unacceptable levels.

Research into creatine is in its infancy. While everything that we have learned to date indicates that the proper use of creatine is safe, there's still a lot we need to learn about this natural nutrient. For the latest updates, visit the web site: www.raysahelian.com.

CHAPTER 5

MUSCLES MADE SIMPLE

In order to fully understand how creatine works, it's important to know what muscles are made of and how they function. While muscle movement may seem like a simple action, it is actually the result of a complex series of chemical and biomechanical events. Creatine assists in this process by providing a source of fuel for immediate muscle contraction. But creatine cannot make muscles move on its own, any more than gasoline can move a car without an engine. It takes a lot more than fuel to produce the intricate and controlled movements that allow us to lift weights, sprint, and perform all other physical endeavors. Without creatine, however, your muscles would run out of "steam" in less than ten seconds, so it obviously plays a vital role in muscle contraction and strength development. In this chapter, we'll give you an overview of some of these biomechanical events, and look at how creatine fits into this larger picture.

Use It or Lose It

A friend of ours was hospitalized recently. He is a 52-year-old active walker, who often goes on hiking trips. He has well-developed calf muscles and thick thighs. Unfortunately, he came down with a severe case of pneumonia and ended up in the hospital. Things took a turn for the worse. None of the antibiotics seemed to be killing the germs causing the infection. His fever rose to 105 degrees, his lungs filled with fluid, and he ended up on a respirator. We visited him daily. Within two weeks the muscles of his legs shriveled to the size of someone who had never worked out. It was sad to see this change. During the third week, his infection came under control, the tubes were removed from his throat, and he was able to sit up in bed. Shortly thereafter, he started walking around his room, and a few days later, left the hospital. He gradually resumed his daily walks, initially for only a block or two, but within one month he was back to his full three-mile walks. He started hiking in the mountains again, and within another two months, his legs and calves were back to their original size.

It's truly amazing how quickly muscles shrink when they're inactive, and how fast they grow when demands are placed upon them!

Muscles and Bones

Muscles allow the body to stand upright and move in a coordinated fashion. Most muscles connect to bones, and the entire network of skeletal muscles and bones is called the bony-lever system. Muscles are connected to the outer coating of the bones by tendons—strong and dense-

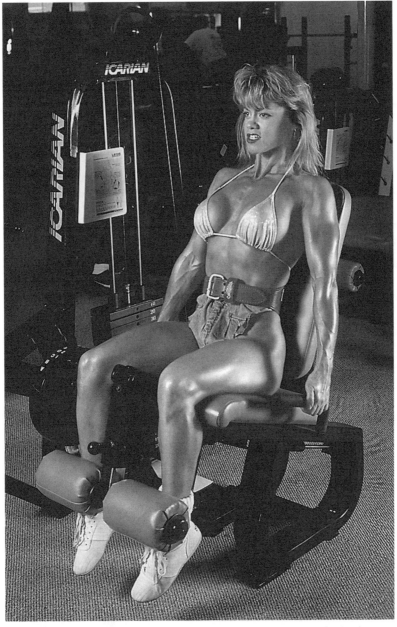

Creatine's ability to boost protein synthesis helps
Marla Duncan increase the size and density
of her muscle fibers.

ly-constructed connective tissues that allow the force of muscle contraction to be transmitted from the muscle cells to the outer reaches of the bones.

The point at which the muscle/tendon connects to the relatively stable part of the skeleton is called the muscle's origin. The point where the muscle/tendon attaches to the bone that performs the movement is known as the insertion. The locations of these origins and insertions are permanent, and cannot be modified through training. Therefore, if a person has genetically short biceps, that muscle trait will always remain. The biceps can increase their size through muscle growth, but they cannot grow outward by changing their connection points to the bones. This is one of the "givens" that we all have to live with.

One important group of skeletal muscles that does not attach to bones is our facial muscles. We use these facial muscles in order to communicate and give a signal to others about our moods. Unlike all other muscles, facial muscles move skin, not bone.

What Muscles Are Made Of

There are more than 430 muscles in the body which permit voluntary motion. While each of these muscles has a specific function, all muscles share common characteristics. Skeletal muscles are made up primarily of water, which accounts for over 75 percent of their weight. Another 20 percent is protein, while the last 5 percent is made up of a variety of inorganic salts and other substances, including minerals, enzymes, fats, carbohydrates, and creatine.

Approximately 95 percent of the body's creatine is found in skeletal muscles. Two-thirds of this is in the

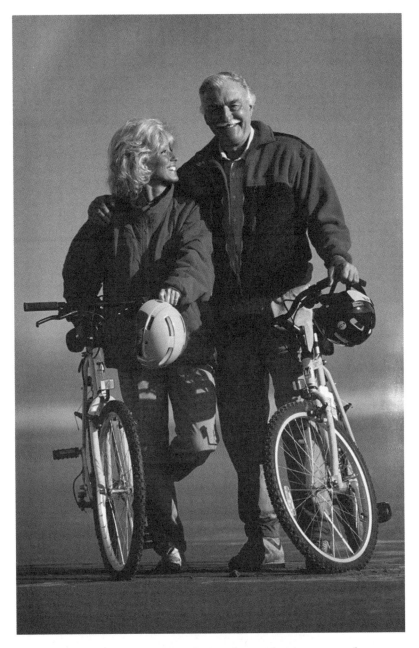

**Creatine builds strength, endurance, and
self-confidence in people of all ages.**

form of creatine phosphate, while the other third is a chemically-unbound form known as free creatine. Older and more sedentary individuals tend to have a higher level of free creatine and less creatine phosphate.

Creatine is not manufactured in the muscles. It either enters the body through the intestines as a dietary nutrient, or it is synthesized in the liver, pancreas, or kidneys. In both cases, it is transported to the walls of the muscle cells by the bloodstream. These muscle cells draw the creatine from the blood and hold on to it until it is needed for energy production. This transport process is virtually one-way. In fact, a 1968 study by Fitch found that creatine concentrations within muscles are 200 times greater than they are in the blood surrounding the muscles.

The Muscle Fiber

Each muscle is covered with fibrous connective tissue that gives it form and helps protect it from injury. There are also several other fibrous tissues within the muscle itself that help in these functions. The basic unit of the muscle is the muscle fiber, which runs lengthwise through the muscle. There are approximately 250 million muscle fibers in the human body. It is the action of these fibers that allows the muscles to contract.

The muscle fiber is not a uniform mass. When viewed at the microscopic level, it is actually a complex assembly of numerous elements. The fiber is made up of many smaller parts called myofibrils, each no larger than a micron (0.00004 inch). Each of the myofibrils, in turn, is comprised of still smaller sub-units called sarcomeres, which are the functional units of the muscle fiber. It is

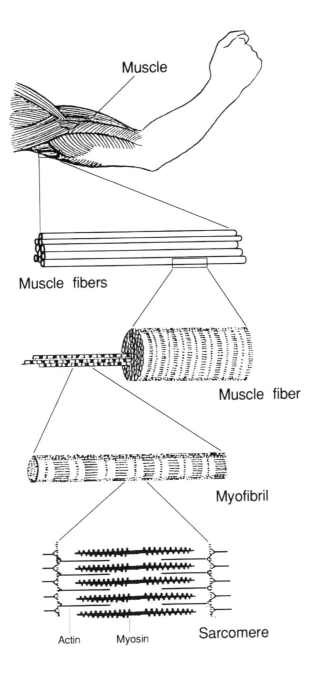

Muscle

Muscle fibers

Muscle fiber

Myofibril

Actin Myosin Sarcomere

Muscle Components

within the sarcomere that the contractile action of the muscle takes place.

There are two types of protein-based myofilaments within the sarcomere: a thin actin filament, and a thicker myosin filament. The actin is attached to the outer edge of the sarcomere, while the myosin is in its center. When viewed from the side, these two filaments appear to be on top of each other, like a layer cake.

The larger myosin filaments have small projections on them called crossbridges. These crossbridges extend from the body of the myosin and, when chemically "excited" in the presence of calcium, connect to the actin filaments at specific receptor sites. The crossbridges then grab onto the actin, much as the hands of a person climbing a rope would. This forces the actin filament towards the center of the sarcomere, while the myosin filament moves toward its outer edge. As a result, the two filaments "slide" past each other, causing a reduction in the length of the sarcomere. This microscopic contraction, when multiplied by the millions of sarcomeres in the muscle fiber (and the thousands of fibers in the entire muscle), is what causes muscle contraction. All muscular movement is caused by this sliding of myofilaments within the sarcomere. Creatine provides much of the initial energy that allows this movement to take place.

Muscle Fiber Types

There are two major types of muscle fibers: fast-twitch (FT) and slow-twitch (ST). Everybody has both types of fibers in their muscles, but the relative amount that a person has of each can vary widely. Some athletes, in fact, have fast- to slow-fiber ratios as high as 8 or 9 to 1, while

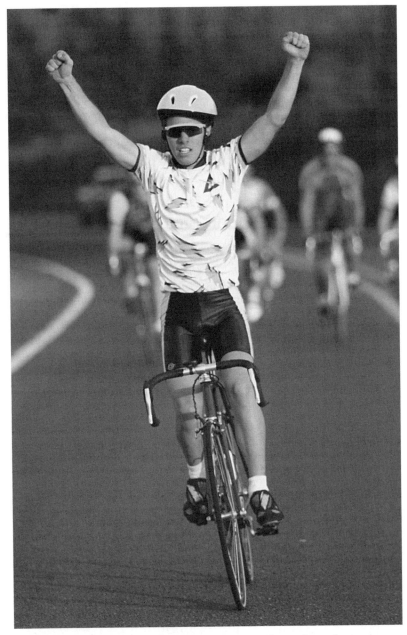

Cyclists find that the power, speed, and endurance they get from creatine enable them to shave precious seconds off of their race times.

most persons have more equal proportions of each. This fiber ratio, which can even vary between the muscles of the same person, is determined by genetics and cannot be altered significantly by training. All muscle fibers, however, respond to athletic training by improving their ability to perform.

Fast-twitch fibers, as their name implies, contract rapidly in response to a stimulus. They also have a great capacity for producing the high-energy compound known as ATP, due to their ability to release calcium quickly during exercise (which aids in speedy muscle contraction). The FT fibers are used almost exclusively for activities which demand a rapid production of power, such as weightlifting and sprinting, and in those situations where stop-and-go movements are required, as in basketball and volleyball. In fact, FT fibers can contract and develop tension twice as quickly as the slow-twitch fibers. The fast-twitch fibers also increase the most in size. This is due to the relatively greater enlargement of their actin and myosin filaments.

Slow-twitch fibers, on the other hand, are called into use when a slow speed of contraction is required. These fibers are well-suited to less intensive aerobic activities because they are relatively resistant to fatigue. They also have a superior ability to produce ATP in conditions where oxygen is available. This ability is due to the greater blood flow in this type of fiber, as well as the larger number of mitochondria (energy factories) within the cells of ST fibers. These fibers also contain a large amount of myoglobin, a reddish-colored compound that helps to store and transport oxygen to the muscle cell. This is why ST fibers are sometimes called red fibers.

Research has shown that fast-twitch fibers have much more creatine than slow-twitch fibers. One study found that the creatine content of the vastus lateralis (thigh) muscle, which is 59 percent FT fibers, is significantly higher than the soleus (calf) muscle, which is 35 percent FT fibers. This makes sense, since fast-twitch fibers are better suited to the quick, immediate movements that are creatine's specialty. Over time, evolution has given us a greater supply of creatine fuel in the muscles where it is most needed.

Improving Your Muscles With Creatine

Our muscles are very elaborate pieces of machinery. While at first glance it may seem uncomplicated, muscle movement is actually the result of an intricate set of chemical and biomechanical actions. Some of these actions are determined by genetics and are beyond your control. But others can be manipulated to increase muscle strength and improve your performance. You can teach your brain to send stronger signals to the muscle, recruiting more and more of your sarcomeres and myofilaments for growth. You can also increase the size and density of your fast- and slow-twitch muscle fibers by training with peak intensity and following a sound program of nutrition that gives your body the raw materials it needs for strength and mass gains. That includes the right amount of creatine, which will give your muscles the additional fuel they need for maximum sports achievement.

CHAPTER 6

HOW MUSCLES
USE ENERGY

Muscle contraction requires energy. Without a continuous supply of this chemical energy, your muscles would run out of "steam" and stop dead in their tracks. As a result, the human body has developed three different ways of coming up with the energy it needs to power muscle movement. This ensures that energy will be available at all times and at a wide variety of intensity levels. Creatine is an essential component of one of these three energy pathways. It allows a compound called ATP (adenosine triphosphate) to be recreated after it has been chemically split apart to produce energy. The reconstituted ATP is then available for additional muscle contractions, allowing you to lift more or move faster than you would otherwise have been able to. In this chapter, we will review these three energy systems and see how they interact to permit smooth and efficient muscle movement.

Getting Energy from Food

All of the energy produced by the body is generated through a series of chemical reactions within the body's tissues. The raw materials for these reactions are the foods we eat: carbohydrates, fats, and proteins. These foods are, by and large, digested in the stomach and assimilated in the intestines. Many go through additional chemical changes in the liver. Some of these broken-down food components are then converted within each cell into ATP, which traps a large portion of the potential energy. These chemical reactions also convert food into glycogen (the storage form of glucose) and the fatty acids that are stored in the body's adipose tissue (commonly called body fat). The remainder is lost as body heat.

Adenosine Triphosphate

Adenosine triphosphate, or ATP, is known as the cell's "energy currency." It is used for building new tissues, nerve transmission, blood circulation, digestion, gland secretions, and, of course, for muscle contraction. Every cell has its own independent supply of ATP. Since it cannot be supplied by the blood or other tissues, each cell must continually recycle ATP using the raw materials available inside and outside the cell.

As its name implies, ATP has three phosphate molecules bonded to an adenosine molecule. When one of the chemical bonds connecting these three phosphate molecules is broken during a reaction known as hydrolysis, a great deal of energy is created. This transfer of energy is called phosphorylation. It is the breaking of bonds between these phosphate molecules that pro-

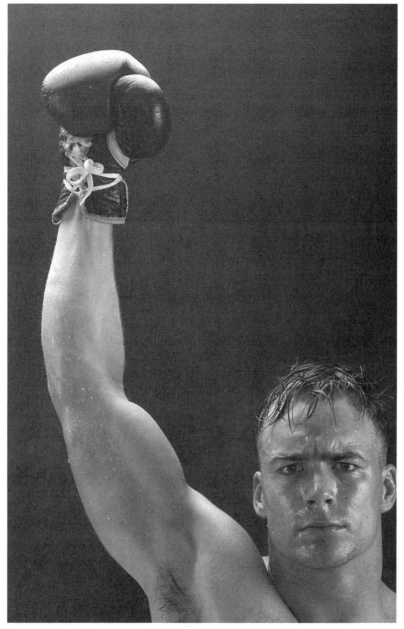

Because creatine provides a longer-lasting source of fuel for muscle movement, boxers maintain more fighting force during their matches.

duces all of the energy utilized by the body. Despite its importance, there is only about 90 grams (three ounces) of ATP in the body at any one time. This is enough to provide maximal energy for less than ten seconds. Therefore, ATP must be constantly resynthesized through a variety of chemical means.

There are three main pathways for the energy production the body needs to live and grow. All involve the use of ATP as the basis for energy production. Two of these pathways are called anaerobic energy systems, which means that the chemical processes producing the energy do not utilize oxygen. They include the ATP-CP system and glycolysis. The third pathway utilizes oxygen in its chemical reactions and is referred to as the aerobic system.

The ATP-CP System

This system is used as the immediate source of energy for the body. Activities such as weight training, sprinting, powerlifting, and the martial arts, which require rapid and immediate energy for maximal performance, are heavily dependent on the ATP-CP system. This system involves an exchange of energy between two molecules, ATP and CP (creatine phosphate). When one of the three phosphate bonds in ATP is chemically broken, a great deal of energy is released. This activates specific sites on the actin and myosin myofilaments of the muscle fiber, producing a muscular contraction. This chemical process is enhanced by an enzyme called creatine kinase, which speeds up (catalyzes) the reaction to allow more energy to be produced within a given time frame. Creatine kinase is not altered chemically during this process.

$$ATP \rightarrow ADP + P + Energy$$
$$ADP + CP \rightarrow ATP + C$$

After ATP loses its phosphate molecule, the remaining compound is called ADP (adenosine diphosphate). In some circumstances, one of the two remaining phosphate molecules in ADP is broken off to produce a third compound called AMP (adenosine monophosphate). Usually, however, ADP combines with creatine phosphate (CP). Creatine phosphate is known as the cell's phosphate reservoir. It returns to ADP the phosphate molecule that it lost when it was converted from ATP. This process results in a new ATP molecule and free (chemically unbound) creatine. The ATP-CP system then begins again, with ATP being broken down to ADP for energy. This procedure goes on constantly at the start of physical work, and continues as long as there is CP available to permit the reconstruction of ATP. When your supply of creatine phosphate runs out, this energy pathway grinds to a halt.

The amount of CP in your muscles before excercise is usually greater than the quantity of ATP present. A recent study by Maughan found that CP levels are normally three to four times higher than the available supply of ATP. This CP comprises two-thirds of the cell's total creatine concentration at rest. The other third is in the free (unbound) form. After exercise stops, much of the free creatine produced during exercise recombines with a phosphate molecule to form CP by means of an oxygen-dependent process within the mitochondria of the cell. Creatine kinase speeds up this recovery process. Slow-twitch muscle fibers are able to resynthesize CP quicker than fast-twitch fibers because of their higher aerobic potential and the lower level of lactic acid in these fibers following exercise.

A study by Soderlund found that our muscles replenish half of the depleted CP within one minute after a short workout. In five minutes, most, but not all, of the CP that existed prior to exercise has been restored. So creatine functions as an energy bank, helping your muscles to fuel their contractions, and then restoring your energy supplies after exercise has ceased. You can think of it as making a withdrawal from your savings account to pay the rent and later replenishing the bank account with your paycheck.

However, not all of the available free creatine gets converted to CP. Part of this creatine gets broken down into a waste product called creatinine, which is then excreted in the urine. The 1994 Balsom article reports that approximately two grams of creatinine is produced by a sedentary 155 pound (70 kilogram) man each day. In fact, one of the routine blood tests done by doctors is to check for creatinine levels. When they are elevated, a doctor suspects kidney damage, because a normally functioning kidney can easily excrete lots of creatinine. As we age, we tend to have less muscle mass, so the average rate of creatinine excretion declines.

The main advantage of the ATP-CP energy system is that it can go to work immediately, something that the other energy systems can't do. If it weren't for this system, we would be unable to sprint, lift heavy weights, or do any other work which requires immediate full effort. Track-and-field events would start in slow motion. ATP-

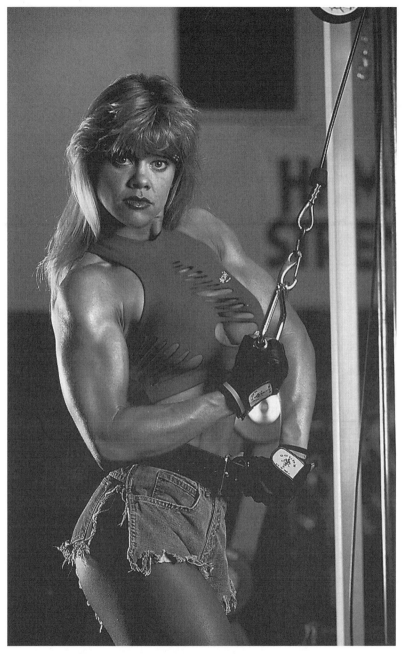

**Marla Duncan has seen dramatic progress in her
definition and vascularity while using creatine.**

CP, therefore, fills the gap between the start of exercise and the times when the other two energy systems kick in.

Glycolysis

The second anaerobic system is glycolysis. This system provides most of the energy for medium-duration activities. During glycolysis, a glucose molecule enters the cell from the blood and is transformed into pyruvic acid through a series of complex reactions involving ATP. These reactions allow a significant amount of energy to be produced quickly for muscular contraction, just as the ATP-CP system begins to slow down. Glycolysis can also use muscle glycogen (the storage form of glucose) and the glycerol formed when a fat molecule is broken down as its initial raw material for energy production.

Lactic acid is a by-product of glycolysis. In the absence of adequate oxygen (anaerobic conditions), the pyruvic acid is converted into lactic acid and alanine, which actually helps keep glycolysis going by removing excess hydrogen ions that would normally grind it to a halt. The lactic acid escapes into the bloodstream and away from the muscle. This escape mechanism is only temporary, however, because the levels of lactic acid in the blood and muscle eventually rise. This increased acidity inactivates some of the enzymes used in glycolysis, which reduces the ability of the muscles to contract. Fatigue sets in and exercise must stop.

Creatine actually delays the point at which this acidity reaches a critical level. That is because creatine phosphate increases the muscle's buffering capacity, helping the individual cell to resist the changes in acidity. If it weren't for creatine phosphate, the glycolytic energy pathway would stop even earlier. The greater the supply of creatine phosphate, the longer it can assist the muscle cells as a buffer.

Lactic acid is usually considered to be a waste product, an unfortunate part of working out that we all must live with. This is not the case. Lactic acid is actually a valuable source of chemical energy that is stored by the body during exercise until sufficient oxygen is available. In the presence of adequate oxygen, lactic acid is converted back into pyruvic acid, ready for use as an energy source. Without lactic acid, glycolysis would run into a dead end and fatigue would occur even earlier. Alanine, lactic acid and pyruvic acid can also be converted back into glucose in the liver, providing more raw material for future energy. So, lactic-acid formation is simply part of our body's integrated biological system.

The Aerobic System

The third type of energy production is the aerobic system. This system releases 95 percent of the potential energy in each glucose and fat molecule through a complex set of processes called the Krebs cycle, which can only function in the presence of oxygen. The end product of this cycle is more ATP. This aerobic system makes use of the mitochondria, the principal source of energy within each cell.

It is important to remember that many sports use the two anaerobic energy systems (ATP-CP and glycolysis) to provide most of their energy requirements. Bodybuilding and sprinting, for example, rely on anaerobic systems for virtually all of their energy production.

As a result, you can't burn a lot of fat while lifting weights or running 100-meter dashes, since fat can only be burned when oxygen is available. If you have excess body fat, you should "melt" it away by participating in lower-intensity activities that utilize the aerobic energy pathway, such as walking, biking, in-line skating, and jogging.

How the Three Systems Interact

All three energy systems are interrelated. Rather than switching on and off as the lights of a traffic signal do, the three systems overlap to provide a smooth blending from one means of energy production to another. This allows the body to perform at its best through many different levels of exercise intensity. For example, while submaximal exercise is basically "aerobic" in nature, studies have shown that creatine phosphate levels drop during moderate-intensity cycling, although not as much as they do in sprinting or powerlifting. This shows that the ATP-CP system is recruited to some extent even for so-called aerobic activities.

These interrelationships allow the body to overcome the limitations of each individual energy pathway. The ATP-CP system gets things moving while the glycolytic and aerobic pathways are unable to produce energy, then phases out as the other systems take on more of the load. Athletes can use the knowledge of these interrelationships to their advantage. Everyone is familiar with the burning sensation that comes from high levels of lactic acid in the muscle. This acidity, in fact, is the most common reason why muscle movement grinds to a halt. Creatine supplementation allows you to keep the ATP-CP system going longer, which keeps lactic-acid levels lower than they would have been otherwise, for a greater period of time. This permits a net increase in the amount of work completed, helping you to achieve your athletic goals.

The Vital Role of Creatine

Creatine plays a vital role in producing the energy needed for muscle contraction. As we have seen, creatine phosphate permits the resynthesis of ATP, which allows more energy to be generated through the ATP-CP system. The enzyme creatine kinase also speeds up this process. So creatine boosts your muscles' energy through two different types of chemical reactions. This makes it even more important that you have adequate supplies of this nutrient within your muscle cells. Only then will you be able to take full advantage of the power of creatine to maximize your strength and sports performance.

CHAPTER 7

BENEFITS FOR ATHLETES

C reatine has the power to help athletes in many different sports, and can also help non-athletes who want to look more muscular. Because it is an essential component in one of the body's main energy systems, creatine is able to boost muscular strength and increase the speed of explosive movements. It also promotes increases in lean body mass, which can be a distinct advantage in a number of sports. The ways in which creatine helps athletes, however, depend on the specific activity. Here we will discuss how this wonderful supplement can boost performance in a variety of sports. We will also look at other health-related benefits that scientists have recently discovered.

Bodybuilding

Bodybuilders were among the first athletes to discover creatine. Bodybuilders have two main objectives in their sport: increasing muscular size and reducing body fat levels to permit greater definition and vascularity. Creatine helps on both counts. Virtually all bodybuilding movements are fueled by the two anaerobic energy pathways: ATP-CP and glycolysis. Since glycolysis produces lactic acid, which eventually makes the muscle fibers so acidic that muscular movement must stop, it's best to keep the body in the ATP-CP system for as long as possible. This enables the bodybuilder to achieve the greatest work output and the highest level of exercise intensity.

Creatine supplementation loads the muscle cells with as much raw material for ATP resynthesis as possible. It also promotes greater nitrogen retention and protein synthesis by increasing intracellular water levels. Bodybuilders are then able to achieve progressive resistance in their weight training. Provided that the athlete gives his or her body the other raw materials for muscle growth (such as amino acids, vitamins, and minerals), and gets adequate recuperation to permit full recovery from the stresses of training, the end result will be greater muscular strength and an increase in lean muscle mass.

Creatine also seems to lower body fat levels. About a third of our survey respondents mentioned reduced body fat as a benefit from creatine use. While the reason for these improvements is still unclear, it appears to relate to the higher energy expenditure produced by the increases in training volume and total muscle mass. (You burn more calories each day just keeping that extra muscle alive and well!) These gains in definition and vascularity are highly prized in bodybuilding, where competitive athletes often step on stage with body fat levels as low as three percent.

Powerlifting

Powerlifters train in order to lift as much weight as possible. There are three competitive events in powerlifting:

bench press, deadlift, and squat. Each event requires the athlete to perform a single repetition of a movement, which is an action powered exclusively by the ATP-CP system. Powerlifters use creatine to maximize their ability to manufacture ATP quickly and under very demanding circumstances. This intensifies their explosiveness and muscular strength. Creatine's ability to enhance protein synthesis also boosts the number of myofilaments within the muscle fibers, which leads to additional gains in muscular power over time. Creatine-induced gains in muscle mass, while not considered in the judging criteria for the sport, may nevertheless help to "psych out" competitors when they approach the lifting platform. However, as noted in our profile of the Gold's Powerlifting Team, mass increases can sometimes push you over the weight limit and into another class. As a result, size gains (and creatine dosages) may need to be tailored to an athlete's specific situation.

Track and Field

Track and field athletes were some of the earliest users of creatine. Competitive use of this supplement has been reported as far back as the 1992 Barcelona Olympics. An article in the London *Times* reported that gold medalist Linford Christie had used creatine for his 100-meter win. Sally Gunnell, who won the gold medal in the 400-meter hurdles, was another creatine user. Since 1992, the use of creatine in this sport has exploded.

With maximal ATP resynthesis, a sprinter can run faster for a longer period of time under certain circumstances. These short-distance events also place a premium on explosiveness and immediate reaction to the starting gun, so creatine's ability to promote virtually instantaneous responses to the body's energy demands can provide a competitive advantage.

A 1993 study by Harris found that creatine supplementation reduced running times for athletes who performed four bouts of a 300-meter sprint with three minutes of rest in between. The average 1.5-second reduction in mean running time was most pronounced on the final 300 meters. The increases in speed were even greater when the runners did four bouts of a 1,000-meter sprint with four minutes of rest in between. The mean running time dropped by a total of 13.0 seconds for the four bouts, and by 5.5 seconds during the last bout. The test subjects took a total of 30 grams of creatine along with 30 grams of glucose per day for six days.

On the other hand, a 1997 study by Terrillion found no such improvement in performance when there was 60 minutes between bouts. Terrillion measured the running times of twelve competitive male runners in two 700-meter races, then gave six of them 20 grams of creatine for five days to see what effect supplementation had on their speeds. There was no significant difference between the creatine and placebo groups. It appears that ATP stores are fully recovered within 60 minutes even without creatine, so supplementation provides no benefit in this situation.

For longer races creatine use may not be beneficial. Although creatine should theoretically help buffer the buildup of lactic acid that can limit performance during long-distance events, a study by Balsom found that there was actually an increase of 25.8 seconds in the time of a 6,000-meter (6-km) run on a forest track with undulating terrain. Test subjects consumed 20 grams of creatine along with 4 grams of glucose per day for six days. The researchers suggested that the average 2-lb (0.9-kg) increase in the body mass of the creatine users may have been responsible for the drop in performance. This appears to have negated the strength and buffering effects of the supplement. The precise trade-off distance where creatine use is no longer advisable has yet to be determined.

Creatine may also improve performance in the javelin, discus, and shot-put. These events place a high value on explosive movement, which is fueled almost exclusively by the ATP-CP energy pathway. The added strength and power that these athletes would get from creatine should therefore allow them to throw their projectiles further and with greater consistency, particularly during repeated bouts. No studies on these events have been published to date.

Creatine may not improve performance in the broad and high jumps, however, because in these events the body is moving through the air most of the time. Since creatine-induced gains in strength and speed cannot help the athlete while he or she is in the air, the weight gains usually stimulated by the supplement may prove to be the dominant factor in determining overall performance and competitive standing.

Boxing and the Martial Arts

In boxing and the martial arts, the ability to maintain repeated punching is the most significant gain. These ongoing increases in explosive power and speed are even more important than the extensive strength gains from the supplement. All of these explosive movements are fueled by the ATP-CP system. Creatine could enable boxers and martial artists to surprise their opponents by moving with greater speed and hitting with more force. This would let creatine users establish dominance in the ring or on the mat from the beginning, helping to defeat their adversaries psychologically. Creatine has an even greater impact in latter rounds. Because the supplement provides a longer-lasting source of fuel for muscle movement, boxers and martial artists maintain more of their punching power during the match, while their competitors lose strength and fighting force with each passing minute. These higher energy levels enable athletes to keep on throwing punches or kicks at their demoralized opponents. This ability to postpone the onset of fatigue is crucial in these demanding events.

Volleyball, Tennis, and Other Racquet Sports

In volleyball and the racquet sports, athletes must serve the ball at maximum velocity, and then respond rapidly to their opponent's actions. These movements are heavily dependent on the ATP-CP energy pathway. When you can repeatedly put the ball over the net at greater speed, your competitor will have to react quicker and work harder to return the serve. This may catch him or her off-guard and establish a psychological advantage. At the very least, it will tire out your adversary sooner. Responding to a serve also requires bursts of explosive power, both during the sprint to arrive at the correct position for a volley and during the arm and body movements that send the ball over the net at maximum speed. Tennis and volleyball players also try to fool their competitors by maintaining a body stance which suggests a particular direction for their next action. They hold this stance until the last possible moment, then surprise their opponents by making a split-second change in position. These explosive movements are all maximized through creatine supplementation. Creatine also increases an athlete's endurance. This can be a significant benefit, particularly at the professional level where matches can last several hours.

Benefits for Other Sports

Creatine will likely provide benefits for athletes in other sports as well. These include wrestling, football, basketball, soccer, hockey, swimming, rowing, and cycling. Creatine's ability to increase muscular strength and endurance is often cited as the biggest advantage for these sports. Clearly, if athletes are stronger, they can escape from wrestling holds with greater ease or tackle with more force. Prolonged endurance also allows these athletes to remain in peak condition for more playing time. The increased muscle mass provided by creatine helps in wrestling as well, where the ability to use the body's weight can be instrumental in forcing an adversary onto the mat for a pin. Added muscle helps football players block their opponents in the lineup, too.

Many athletes benefit from the increased sprinting speed and explosive power that creatine permits. Basketball players often move explosively in their attempts to outsmart the other team and shoot the ball into the hoop. When they recover the ball and break for the other end of the court, their ability to dribble and sprint quickly is often decisive in determining the winning team. Soccer and hockey players also combine sprinting with explosive movements as they strive to maneuver past their opponents and make the goal. Competitive swimmers, rowers, and cyclists find that the power, speed, and endurance that creatine provides enable them to shave precious seconds off of their times, which can catapult them to victory in their activities. As with track and field athletes, the greatest benefits occur during events of shorter duration .

A 1996 study by Rossiter has confirmed these performance gains for rowers. A five-day period of creatine supplementation improved rowing speeds by 2.3 seconds, or just over 1 percent, during a 1,000 meter event. While the athletes using creatine always rowed faster than those taking the placebo, the differential between the two groups increased as the event progressed. During the final 400 meters of the race, creatine users had significantly greater speeds than those taking the "sugar pill." Rossiter found that creatine increased the power production of these competitive rowers instead of changing their stroke rate. He attributed these improvements in part to the buffering capacity of creatine, which rose approximately 3 percent as a result of supplementation. The creatine dose in this study was 0.25 grams per kilogram of bodyweight (17.5 grams for a 70 kg or 155 lb athlete).

Swimmers improve their performance with creatine as well. Several members of the U.S. swim team at the 1996 Summer Olympics reportedly used the supplement to increase their times. A study presented at the International Conference on Overtraining in Sport by a research team headed by Dr. Rick Kreider of the University of Memphis also found significant improvements in sprint times with creatine supplementation. Eighteen male and female competitive swimmers took 21 grams of creatine and 4.2 grams of maltodextrin per day for 9 days. Compared to the control group, the creatine users had reductions of 0.27 seconds, 0.93 seconds and 0.36 seconds for the first, second and third 100-meter bouts, respectively. There were 60 seconds of rest between each bout. "This resulted in a cumulative gain of 3.1 meters over their counterparts, enough to provide a clear competitive edge," noted Dr. Kreider. "There were also improvements of 4.8 percent in mean total work and 4.9 percent in average power for the three sprint tests." However, a study by Thompson did not find an improvement in exercise performance when female athletes took 2 grams of creatine per day for six weeks. There was no effect on muscle creatine concentration or muscle metabolism at this low dosage, either. A loading phase or higher daily dosage is therefore required to achieve the desired performance benefits in swimmers.

Health Benefits of Creatine

While this chapter has focused on the sports-related advantages for athletes, recent research has shown that creatine provides other health benefits as well. A 1996 study by Dr. Earnest found that fifty-six days of creatine supplementation produced a 6 percent reduction in total cholesterol levels in the blood. This reduction continued for four weeks after creatine use stopped before returning to their original levels. The results for triglycerides (fatty acids) and very-low-density lipoprotein are even better: Levels of these blood components dropped by 23 percent after four weeks of creatine supplementation and remained 26 percent below their original levels four weeks after the test subjects were taken off creatine. Blood levels for other lipoproteins were unaffected during this experiment. These findings are intriguing, and offer new possibilities for research with creatine.

Creatine has been proven effective in treating gyrate atrophy, an eye disease characterized by night blindness, constriction of visual fields, and myopia (nearsightedness). It is caused by low levels of an enzyme involved in the breakdown of the amino acid ornithine. Untreated, the disease can lead to total blindness in thirty to forty years. A dosage of 1.5 grams of creatine monohydrate per day for one year was shown to reduce the symptoms of this disease in nearly all patients studied. No side effects were reported other than a 10 percent weight gain, presumably lean muscle mass.

Creatine supplementation also reverses the effects of GAMT (guanidinoacetate methyltransferase) deficiency. The inefficiency or failure of this metabolic pathway can impair the development of motor control and thought processes in infants. One report published on a 22-month infant found that 4 grams of creatine monohydrate per day for twenty-five months brought substantial clinical improvement, including more controlled movements and the disappearance of several brain abnormalities. Supplementation produced normal concentrations of creatine in the brain and body.

Creatine may also benefit AIDS patients and elderly individuals with muscle-wasting syndrome. Since creatine promotes protein synthesis and facilitates increases in lean muscle mass, this supplement is currently being investigated as a way to counteract the impacts of disease and the aging process. It could also be utilized to assist persons whose muscles have atrophied due to injury or extended illness.

CHAPTER 8

INTERVIEW WITH AN EXPERT

C onrad P. Earnest, Ph.D., is one of the pioneers of creatine research. He has completed five studies on this supplement, ranging from its impact on peak anaerobic power and muscular strength to its effect on cholesterol and lipid levels in the blood. The results of these studies have been published in either abstract or article form in 13 different journals, including *Medicine and Science in Sports and Exercise* and *Clinical Science*. He completed his doctoral studies in kinesiology at Texas Women's University in Denton, Texas. His specialization is in exercise physiology, with a secondary emphasis on nutrition and food science. Conrad Earnest holds bachelor's and master's degrees from the University of Akron, Ohio. He is also Manager and Director of Research and Staff Development for Goodbody's Fitness Clinic in Dallas, Texas.

**Q: How did you first get involved in
creatine research?**

A: Several years ago, one of my bodybuilder friends told
me about creatine. He said he had tried it and gotten
very good results. Frankly, I was skeptical. Everything in the world gets shoved at bodybuilders. And
if there's even a hint of rationale for it working,
chances are they'll take it. That really gets weary after
a while. I have people who approach me all the time,
saying that I should try this or that. I'll ask where it's
been shown to do anything, and typically the answer
is they don't have a clue.

After I heard about creatine, I went to my University Medical School and read one of the early studies.
That stirred my curiosity. At the time, very few people
were interested in doing research on creatine. I knew
physiologically that it made sense, but then, so do
many things. Sometimes, a study shows that something works intravenously, but may not be effective
when taken orally. Digestion is a whole new beast. So
I decided to find out for sure.

After I completed my initial study, I knew that
creatine worked. So I got more and more involved in
research on this supplement. I've now done five studies, the results of which have been published in either
abstract or article form in 13 different journals. I plan
to do a lot more creatine research in the future.

**Q: Is the evidence on creatine really that
convincing?**

A: The data on creatine is becoming abundantly clear. It
definitely works. Now, I won't stand up and say that it

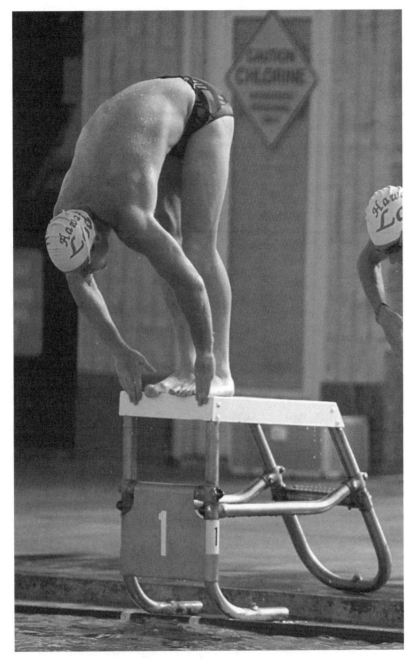

**The explosive power swimmers get from creatine
gives them a competitive edge during their meets.**

will work for every individual, but then, nothing works for everyone. Creatine has gotten the attention of a lot of people in the exercise-physiology community who are very well respected. There's no doubt about it.

Q: Athletes in which sports will benefit from creatine supplementation?

A: Creatine will improve performance in any sport where there is an explosive or fatigue element. This includes bodybuilding, powerlifting, swimming, the martial arts, volleyball, tennis, and sports that require sprinting. The potential for gains is really far-reaching. Creatine reduces recovery time and increases the amount of cumulative work you can perform. And that's what training is all about. If you can do more bouts of work based on your improved recovery, then at the end of the day you will have placed more demands on your muscle. If you also get the appropriate amount of rest, you'll be a better athlete by the time your competition rolls around.

This applies to many different sports. Look at the Olympics. Creatine will help sprinters in all track events up to 800 meters (and maybe as long as 1,600 meters). It will also be of benefit to athletes in sports that involve short sprints such as soccer, basketball, rowing, and cycling. For example, in sprint cycling, you play cat and mouse for three laps and then go for hell on the last lap. That puts a lot of demands on your ATP-CP energy pathway. On the other hand, it's doubtful that creatine will help someone win a marathon. However, it could help them in their training when they do repeats or interval laps.

There is a large group of pre-Olympic swimmers in the Dallas area who are using creatine for sprint events. One 14-year-old improved his time by a full second in the 100-meter race. His mother, who teaches biochemistry, wouldn't let him use creatine for the longest time because of her concerns about supplementation. She is still skeptical, but a bit more open-minded. The results are very far-reaching. The greatest gains are found in shorter distance events.

In boxing and the martial arts, the ability to maintain repeated punching is the most important gain. This explosive power (as opposed to strength) is particularly crucial in the martial arts. These movements are fueled by ATP-CP. If you look at the studies on performance, it shows that creatine may not have much of an effect on the first bout of exercise, but it definitely has an impact on later bouts. So, although your first punch may not have more power, if you're throwing lots of punches, you'll probably have more power at the end of the match. With creatine you'll be able to sustain your energy level better, and prevail while your opponent is fatiguing more quickly.

Tennis players will also benefit. If you can put the ball over the net repeatedly with quicker speed, it will be harder for your opponent to return it. Again, we are looking at the fatigue/recovery aspect. Creatine will also help you sprint and return the balls that your opponent sends your way. At Wimbledon, they play three- to five-hour matches. What would happen if the athletes took a creatine and glucose drink after two hours? Would it increase their performance? Now, that would be an interesting study.

Q: What dosages do you recommend?

A: After a five-day loading sequence at 20 grams per day, 5 to 10 grams a day is all you need to maintain. The exact maintenance dose depends on your exercise intensity and muscle mass. Once you've filled your body's creatine-storage capacity, it's not essential that you take it everyday. You might even skip it on the days you don't work out, since you will use less on those days. Some of the existing research shows that creatine remains in your system for weeks. Once it gets into the muscle, it appears to stay there for a long time. How long, we aren't exactly sure.

I've found that it's best to take creatine before and after a workout. My training is much better when I have half of my creatine dose in a glucose drink 30-40 minutes before I exercise. But it's good to take it afterwards as well, since the most sensitive time for glucose uptake is within an hour after exercise. Therefore, to fully replenish your creatine stores, it makes sense to divide your maintenance dosage in two. Also, protein uptake increases in the hour after exercise when the necessary amino acids are present, so it's important to get in some amino acids during that time period, too.

Q: What should I mix my creatine with?

A: You should always take your creatine with a carbohydrate drink, preferably one that has glucose polymers, dextrose, or maltodextrin in it. The early studies used glucose, but that was only to cover the taste of the creatine so the study participants wouldn't

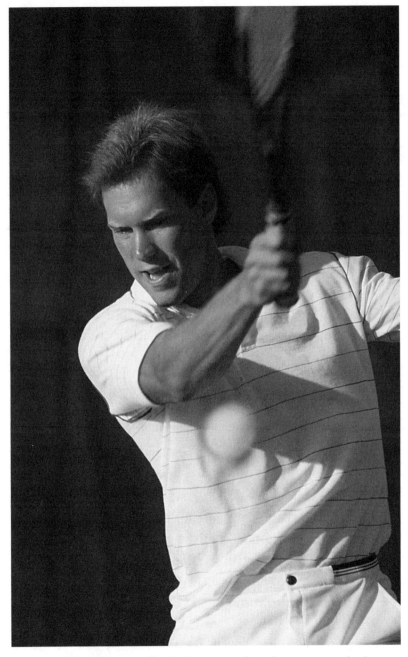

**Tennis players find that creatine increases their
endurance while reducing their reaction time.**

know if they were getting the placebo or not. In any case, the amount of glucose they received in these studies wasn't enough to have an insulin-boosting effect.

Try not to take your creatine with water alone. Fruit juice is a better choice, although the fructose in these juices does not cause as much insulin release as the carbs found in sports drinks with glucose polymers, dextrose, or maltodextrin. For optimal creatine uptake, mix 5 grams of creatine with 30-50 grams of one of these carbs.

Don't drink your creatine with coffee or tea. A study on caffeine and creatine showed that caffeine eliminated the gains in torque production which creatine normally provides. You also want to stay away from soda pop. When you add creatine to soda, it fizzes up big-time, so there's a definite reaction. The people I know who took it this way were pretty miserable for a while. Sports drinks are much better.

Q: Do I need to cycle creatine?

A: I personally think that it's a good idea to periodically stop taking creatine for two to three weeks, and then reload. But that's just a hunch on my part, since there is no research on the subject. Your body gets accustomed to anything after a while. Going off creatine will allow your body to readjust toward its pre-supplementation level. But it's not as if you're washing it out of your system, since creatine remains in your body for at least three to four weeks. I just feel that cycling may facilitate creatine upload in the long term.

There are many questions that are still unanswered about creatine. What is the downstream effect of stopping the body's own production of creatine? We don't know. Recent research from our lab has shown that creatine lowers cholesterol and lipid levels in the blood, which no one would have suspected a year or two ago. So what else does it do? When you supplement, you're playing with the body's natural ability to do something, which may mean "down-regulating" an existing system. So it pays to be cautious. From a philosophical perspective, cycling may be good idea. If the body produces something, it's probably a good idea to let it produce it from time to time. But no one knows for sure. We just don't have all the answers.

Q: What are the long-term benefits of creatine use?

A: Creatine will help athletes in the long term by increasing their overall energetic performance. Creatine improves recovery time, which will help your training. After all, training is a long-term commitment. You're in the gym on a regular basis, always striving to achieve your goals. Creatine will reduce your recuperation time and boost your ability to do work. So the overall change in these training parameters during a two- to three-year period should be much greater than that indicated in the 28-day time frame used in the scientific studies.

The Greenhaff study showed that creatine lowered plasma ammonia levels, which would indicate ATP sparing and better short-term recovery. So far there has been no study on creatine's ability to improve recuperation in the sense of reducing or eliminating delayed-onset muscle soreness. Unfortunately, there are only a handful of people doing studies on creatine, although others are now getting into the act. We are in the forefront of creatine research. Ten to fifteen years from now we will have the answers to a lot of these questions.

Q: Does everyone get the same response from creatine supplementation?

A: No. The response varies. There are also non-responders. Some people can take creatine and it will not improve their performance, apparently because their muscles can't absorb the additional nutrient. No one knows why, but it may be related to insulin sensitivity. Also, if a person's creatine-uptake mechanism is desensitized for some reason, that could also impact the change in performance. However, at this point we don't know enough about this uptake mechanism to determine how to promote maximum sensitivity. Also, there's no research on the percentage of athletes who don't respond to creatine loading. It's all too new, one of many things we don't know.

Q: What's the maximum gain I can get from creatine?

A: That's the $64,000 question. If you take creatine, will your progress continue at the same pace, or increase at an exponential rate? Will you reach a certain point and then stabilize? We don't know. A lot of the answer has to do with mechanisms we currently know nothing about. For thirty-five years, we have been researching carbohydrate metabolism, and we're still discovering things!

Is there a limit to the gains you can achieve? Probably, but then there's a limit to everything. This limit will largely be determined by your storage capacity. But other factors may come into play: the physiological makeup of the cell, protein considerations, amino-acid combinations, the need for adequate glucose, effects on lipids, etc. Future research will reveal some of these things from a molecular standpoint.

There's also the genetic factor. If you take a genetically-gifted athlete and give him or her creatine, he or she will be a better genetically-gifted athlete. Athletes who aren't as genetically gifted can use all the creatine they want, but they probably won't catch up. Now, we could get into a philosophical discussion about supplementation in general but, in the real world, people will use whatever they can (usually within reason) to enhance their performance. Someday it may wind up that everyone will use creatine and nothing will change in terms of placings. The level of competition will just jump a notch. But if you can win in the meantime, I'm sure you won't mind.

Q: Will creatine give me more muscle definition?

A: I'm not sure, to be honest. The data indicate that there might be an effect, but it's probably a secondary impact. I don't want to go out on a limb. To the extent that your lean body mass increases, you will need a modest increase in calories to sustain that added muscle. It won't be a big change, but there would be some effect. Provided that you don't increase your caloric consumption to compensate, this change in the balance between caloric intake and expenditure would lower your body fat level. Your basal metabolic rate could also rise as a result of your exercise program, but once again, the number of calories you burn is a function of your muscle mass. Creatine-induced increases in training volume would also boost your energy expenditure, since you could train longer before fatigue sets in. At the same time, creatine works at least in part because of its ability to increase the effectiveness of insulin. Creatine appears to enhance the uptake of glucose into muscle, so you may wind up with fewer fatty acids circulating in your blood. That could reduce your body fat level to a limited extent.

Q: Does creatine increase the need for protein?

A: That's also unknown at this point. Some studies have suggested that creatine increases protein synthesis by activating specific receptors on the actin and myosin myofilaments. This could be one of the mechanisms for the increase in muscle mass. However, studies of less than ten days indicate that most of the initial gain is probably intracellular water weight. This is understandable, since there really isn't time for appreciable protein synthesis in this short time period. Longer-term studies may show more myofilament formation or an increase in the thickness of the actin and myosin strands, since protein synthesis occurs at a greater rate when there is a high amount of water inside the cell. So if you can increase your intracellular fluid volumes, you may significantly improve your protein synthesis when adequate amino acid supplies are present. How this translates into the need for additional dietary protein is a big question mark.

Q: Can older individuals and non-athletes be helped by creatine?

A: My next research interest will probably be outside the realm of athletics. I want to look at the clinical-medicine side of things. There are populations who suffer from tissue atrophy. Seniors are currently being given growth-hormone injections to counteract the wasting that often occurs with aging, but these injections have major side effects. Growth hormone impairs glucose metabolism and has other negative consequences. While you can get functional increases in muscle mass and strength with growth hormone, some studies have shown that the improvement is the same as that achieved with weight training alone. Yet creatine may help seniors to lead longer, healthier lives.

There is also the AIDS population. Will there be a big increase in muscle mass from creatine supplementation in persons with full-blown AIDS? Will creatine's ability to increase protein synthesis reduce the wasting syndrome? These are the populations we should now address with creatine research. We need to find out how it can help maintain the health of a wide range of individuals in our society.

Q: Do you use creatine yourself?

A: I've used it off and on for more than a year, but it's not a daily thing. I went from 175 to 185 pounds while on creatine, but I also beefed up my weight training and cut out my cardiovascular training at the same time. So it's hard to say exactly what caused what. Now that I've added a 45-minute, high-intensity, stationary bike workout to my training, my strength has stayed up but my weight has dropped back down to 182 pounds. I'm a lot leaner, but that's probably due to the increased cardiovascular exercise and not the creatine. My strength has plateaued, but since I'm juggling so many balls now, including my research projects, that's probably not too surprising. There's only so much time in the day. Still, people at the gym have noticed the change, so I can't complain. The most important thing for me as an exercise physiologist is trying to figure out why creatine works, instead of getting it to work miracles for me.

CHAPTER 9

TOP TEN THINGS YOU SHOULD KNOW ABOUT CREATINE

T his book has provided you with an in-depth look at creatine. This fascinating nutrient has received an increasing amount of attention in the 1990s as scientists have discovered its true potential for boosting strength, muscle mass, and sports performance. While some supplements have their day in the sun and then fade away, creatine is here to stay. Its benefits have been proven in controlled, scientific studies. Respected journals ranging from *Clinical Science* and *The Journal of Biological Chemistry* to the *International Journal of Sport Nutrition* have published articles on creatine that show its advantages as an ergogenic aid.

Now, even athletes who had become jaded from the hype over some other supplements have become true believers. They have discovered first-hand that creatine works. Bodybuilders have seen their strength and muscle mass increase, helping them gain the size needed to dominate their competition on the posing dais. Sprinters report that the boost in strength that creatine provides lets them run faster and leave their fellow racers in the dust. Martial artists and wrestlers have realized that the explosive fighting movements required for victory in their sports are powered by a creatine-dependent system. The increased energy stores from creatine supplementation therefore permit quicker and stronger reactions to the moves of opponents, helping athletes to anticipate and control their adversaries.

There is so much information about creatine nowadays that it has taken an entire book to discuss it all. Here are the highlights:

- **Creatine allows your muscles to store more energy.**

Your muscles rely on a creatine-dependent energy system known as ATP-CP for quick, explosive movements. Since a muscle can store only enough ATP for less than ten seconds of peak contractions, ATP must be constantly replenished for exercise to continue. Creatine phosphate comes to the rescue, giving up its phosphate molecule to allow ATP to be resynthesized. So creatine acts as an energy reservoir. When you need energy, your muscle taps into this reservoir to get the raw material it needs. The more creatine in your muscles, the more potential energy you have available.

- **Creatine increases strength and power.**

Several researchers have confirmed that creatine boosts muscular strength and power. One study found that thirty days of creatine supplementation produced a 6 percent increase in the average weight that athletes could lift on a set with a single repetition. There was also

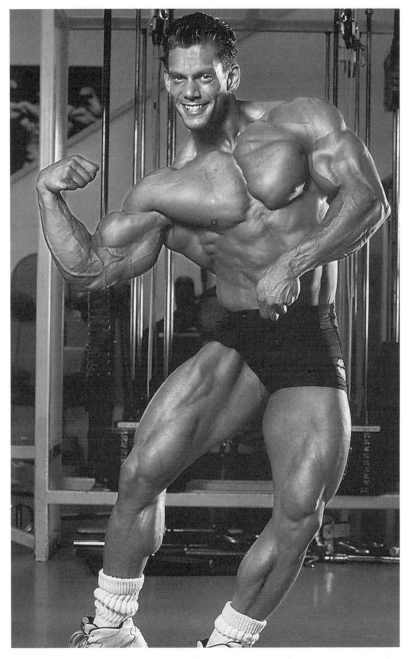

Creatine makes Vince Galanti's muscles feel full of energy and gives them a tremendous pump.

a 43 percent increase in total lifting volume during the month. Another study indicated that persons who took creatine for five days achieved mean power outputs that were 5 percent higher than those using a placebo, while a third study showed an average 5 percent increase in force production during the same time period. So creatine not only makes you stronger, but allows you to work longer and more intensely as well.

- **Creatine boosts protein synthesis and lean muscle mass.**

Greater creatine concentrations within muscles result in additional protein synthesis. This occurs because creatine stimulates the uptake of amino acids in the two contractile proteins of the muscle fiber, known as actin and myosin. The increase in quantity and thickness of these two protein-based myofilaments results in greater muscle mass. Further size gains are stimulated by the enhanced strength and power that creatine provides. This allows you to lift more weight and perform more repetitions, so that you can achieve progressive resistance and consequent muscle growth. These mass increases have been confirmed by three studies, which show average gains of 2.2 to 3.7 pounds (1.0 to 1.7 kilograms) in total body weight within thirty days. That works out to a 2 percent gain in the athletes' average lean muscle mass in one month.

- **While you could get creatine from eating lots of meat, the fat and cholesterol content are major drawbacks.**

Creatine is found in moderate amounts in tuna, cod, salmon, herring, beef, and pork. Tiny amounts are found in milk and even cranberries. Chicken and turkey probably contain creatine as well, but we were unable to document this. It's important to remember that meats and fish contain relatively large amounts of cholesterol. Most meats, especially beef and pork, also contain substantial quantities of fat. Since high cholesterol and fat intake has been linked to heart attacks and other cardiovascular disorders, it's best to avoid eating these foods in large amounts. You should get the creatine you need to improve your strength and power from a creatine monohydrate supplement.

• Your body can only store so much creatine.

There is an upper limit to the amount of creatine your body can store. Studies indicate that no more than 4 grams of creatine can be accumulated in each kilogram of muscle tissue (a bit less than 2 grams per pound of lean muscle mass). Even if you are a vegetarian, you already have some of this creatine supply in your muscles, because your body is able to synthesize it from three amino acids found in food. Meat-eaters have higher creatine concentrations. Your goal should be to fill up (load) your muscles with as much additional creatine as possible, and then keep them as full as you can. Once your creatine stores are saturated, you only need to replace the amount you metabolize during muscle contraction. Any further supplementation simply will be excreted in your urine.

• Once it's in your muscles, creatine stays there for weeks.

While creatine lasts only 1 to 1½ hours in blood plasma, once it enters the muscle fiber it gets "trapped" there for a long time. As a result, creatine concentrations within muscles are 200 times greater than they are in the blood surrounding the muscles. Two studies have shown that creatine levels decline over the course of several weeks, rather than days. So don't worry if you forget to take it for a day or two. A sedentary 155-pound (70-kilogram) man uses up an estimated 2 grams of creatine per day. Scientists recognize that this loss is greater for active persons and athletes with larger muscle mass, but no one knows exactly how much greater. Studies indicate, however, that the creatine levels attained in muscle after a week of loading are maintained for at least four weeks, even with a maintenance dose that is much less than the loading dosage. This is why we recommend a short loading phase and an ongoing maintenance phase.

• Athletes in sports with quick, explosive movements get the most benefit from creatine.

That's because these sports rely most heavily on the ATP-CP system as an energy source. Bodybuilders and power-lifters benefit because creatine helps sustain the short, intense bursts of energy that power the repetitions and sets of their weight training. Sprinters are able to run quicker over short distances due to creatine's ability to boost their energy stores and increase ATP resynthesis. Martial artists and wrestlers also benefit from the greater energy and strength that creatine provides for the split-second movements needed to prevail over their opponents. Creatine can help athletes in many other sports as well, since all sports rely on the ATP-CP system to some extent. However, the less dependent a sport is on intense, explosive movements, the less benefit creatine is likely to have.

- **There is yet no scientific evidence that creatine improves performance in long-distance events such as marathons.**

There have been some anecdotal reports that athletes in these sports may benefit, but others feel that creatine either does not help or may actually hurt. The difficulty in these situations appears to center on the increased muscle mass which creatine provides. While it's great if you're a body-builder or wrestler, it can be a detriment if you have to carry all that weight around during a marathon or triathlon. In such cases, there is a tradeoff between the increased strength you get from creatine and the increased muscle mass.

Perhaps athletes competing in long-distance events such as a Tour de France cycling race could consume a gram or two of creatine with the rest of their fluid consumption. Would a small amount of creatine throughout the day give them a competitive edge? This possibility remains to be explored.

- **Creatine has no side effects when used appropriately.**

The only "adverse effect" that has been documented in the scientific literature is an increase in body mass, which is not a problem for most people. The results from our survey, however, indicate that diarrhea occasionally can occur when creatine is consumed in dosages greater than those recommended in this book. The diarrhea goes away when the dosage is reduced. We would also like to mention that the studies which used high dosages of creatine, such as 20 grams per day, were only a month or less in duration. Therefore, we do not fully know the consequences of high-dose, long-term supplementation yet.

- **The amount of creatine you need increases with your muscle mass and exercise intensity.**

All human skeletal muscle contains creatine. While fast-twitch muscle fibers have more creatine, pound for pound, than slow-twitch fibers, every muscle contains a combination of fast- and slow-twitch fibers. So as you gain muscle mass, your maximum storage potential for creatine goes up as well. The amount of creatine you need to replace each day also depends on how much you metabolize during the muscular contractions involved in your sport. Higher-intensity training will "burn off" more of your creatine stores, requiring additional supplies on a regular basis to keep your creatine-supply bin filled to the brim. It's kind of like topping the tank of your car's gasoline supply, while making sure that nothing spills out. Tailoring your creatine intake to your muscle mass and exercise intensity will allow you to get the maximum gains from this powerful nutrient.

Final Commentary

We wish you the best of luck in your training. If you're currently sedentary, we expect that the quick improvements in muscle that you can get from creatine will encourage you to become more physically active. We hope you enjoy the benefits of creatine, and hope that this promising supplement will help you to look and feel your best, regardless of your age.

THE CREATINE CONTROVERSY

"Dietary Supplement Studied in Three Wrestlers' Deaths" was the title of an article published in the December 19, 1997, issue of *USA Today*.

This headline certainly caught our eyes, especially when we read that the alleged culprit was creatine. The article begins, "The Food and Drug Administration is investigating to see whether three deaths of college athletes since November 7 are linked to a dietary supplement billed as a muscle builder."

As we read this article, we couldn't help but think that something was not right about the incrimination of creatine. Over the past few years, Dr. Sahelian has recommended creatine to at least 100 patients, both of us have interviewed hundreds of users, and we have taken creatine ourselves. No serious side effects have been reported. Doing a thorough research of the published newspaper articles, we learned that all three of the wrestlers died the day before their meets, during crash weight-loss workouts in order to qualify for their wrestling weight category. Jeff Reese, a wrestler from the University of Michigan, was the third of the wrestlers to die within a six-week period. He was attempting to lose 12 pounds in a single day. According to the December 18 and 19, 1997, issues of the *Detroit News*, he had not eaten or drunk liquids since the day before. On December 7, under the supervision of an assistant coach, he donned a rubber suit and rode an exercise bicycle for two to three hours in a 92°F room before becoming ill and collapsing. Wrestlers are also known to use diuretics and laxatives to lose body fluids.

ABC's *Prime Time Live* aired a comprehensive segment on January 7, 1998, regarding these three deaths. The investigative reporting by *Prime Time Live* determined that the causes of death were excessive dehydration, hyperthermia and weight loss, along with the possible use of diuretics and laxatives. The body temperature of one wrestler had reached 106° F! Creatine was not mentioned as being involved in these deaths. We also spoke to reporters from *CBS Evening News* and television's *EXTRA* who interviewed the parents of Jeff Reese. They denied that he was taking creatine.

In our opinion, creatine should not be blamed for the loss of these three lives. The tragedies appear to be due to a combination of overzealous prompting by the coaches, along with the unfortunate, stubborn determination of the wrestlers to make a weight category by shedding pounds rapidly.

Creatine is Safe

We are confident that the use of creatine in proper doses is a safe, natural, and rapid way to gain muscle mass. Both of us are continuing our use of this supplement.

REFERENCES

Almada A, Mitchell T, Earnest C. *Impact of chronic creatine supplementation on serum enzyme concentrations.* FASEB 10(3):4567, 1996.

Anderson O. *Creatine propels British athletes to Olympic gold medals: Is creatine the one true ergogenic aid?* Running Research News 9(1):1-5, 1993.

Balsom P, Ekblom B, Soderlund K, Sjodin B, Hultman E. *Creatine supplementation and dynamic high-intensity intermittent exercise.* Scand J Med Sci Sports 3:143-149, 1993.

Balsom P, Harridge S, Soderlund K, Sjodin B, Ekblom B. *Creatine supplementation per se does not enhance endurance exercise performance.* Acta Physiol Scand 149:521-523, 1993.

Balsom P, Soderlund K, Ekblom B. *Creatine in humans with special reference to creatine supplementation.* Sports Med 18(4): 268-280, 1994. This is a great review article from Karolinska Institute and University College of Physical Education and Sports in Stockholm, Sweden.

Balsom P, Soderlund K, Sjodin B, Ekblom B. *Skeletal muscle metabolism during short duration high-intensity exercise: influence of creatine supplementation.* Acta Physiol Scand 154:303-310, 1995.

Birch R, Noble D, Greenhaff P. *The influence of dietary creatine supplementation on performance during repeated bouts of maximal isokinetic cycling in man.* Eur J Appl Physiol 69:268-270, 1994.

Cooke W, Grandjean P, Barnes W. *Effect of oral creatine supplementation on power output and fatigue during bicycle ergometry.* J Appl Physiol 78(2):670-673, 1995.

Delanghe J, De Slypere J, De Buyzere M, Robbrecht J, Wieme R, Vermeulen A. *Normal reference values for creatine, creatinine and carnitine are lower in vegetarians.* Clin Chem 35:1802-3, 1989.

Earnest C, Almada A, Mitchell T. *High-performance capillary electrophoresis-pure creatine monohydrate reduces blood lipids in men and women.* Clin Sci 91: 113-118, 1996.

Earnest C, Almada A, Mitchell T. *Influence of chronic creatine supplementation on hepatorenal function.* FASEB 10(3): 4566, 1996.

Earnest C, Snell P, Rodriguez R, Almada A, Mitchell T. *The effect of creatine monohydrate ingestion on anaerobic power indices, muscular strength and body composition.* Acta Physiol Scan 153:207-209, 1995.

Fitch C, Jellinek M, Mueller E. *Experimental depletion of creatine and phosphocreatine from skeletal muscle.* J Biol Chem 249(4):1060-1063, 1974.

Fitch C, Shields R. *Creatine metabolism in skeletal muscle: creatine movement across muscle membranes.* J Biol Chem 241(15):3611-3614, 1966.

Fitch C, Shields R, Payne W, Dacus J. *Creatine metabolism in skeletal muscle: specificity of the creatine entry process.* J Biol Chem 243(8):2024-2027, 1968.

Gordon A. Hultman E, Kaijser L, Kristjansson S. *Creatine supplementation in chronic heart failure increases skeletal muscle creatine phosphate and muscle performance.* Cardiovascular Research 30:413-418, 1995.

Green A, Hultman E, Macdonald I, Sewell D, Greenhaff P. *Carbohydrate ingestion augments skeletal muscle creatine accumulation during creatine supplementation in humans.* Am J Physiol 271: E821-E826, 1996.

Greenhaff P. *Creatine supplementation: Recent developments.* Br J Sports Med 30: 276-281, 1996.

Greenhaff P. *Creatine and its application as an ergogenic aid.* Int J Sport Nutrition 5:S100-S110, 1995. Excellent review article.

Greenhaff P, Bodin K, Harris R, Hultman E, Jones D, McIntyre D, Soderund K, Turner D. *The influence of oral creatine supplementation on muscle phosphocreatine resynthesis following intense contraction in man.* J Physiol 46:75P, 1993.

Greenhaff P, Casey A, Short A, Harris R, Soderlund K, Hultman E. *Influence of oral creatine supplementation on muscle torque during repeated bouts of maximal voluntary contraction in man.* Clin Sci 84:565-571, 1995.

Harris R, Soderlund K, Hultman E. *Elevation of creatine in resting and exercise muscles of normal subjects by creatine supplementation.* Clin Sci 83:367-74, 1992.

Harris R, Viru M, Greenhaff P, Hultman E. *The effect of oral creatine supplementation on running performance during maximal short-term exercise in man.* J Physiol 467: 74P, 1993.

Hultman E, Soderland K, Timmons J, Cederblad G, Greenhaff P. *Muscle creatine loading in men.* J Appl Physiol 81(1):232-237, 1996.

Korge P. *Factors limiting adenosine triphosphatase function during high intentsity exercise: thermodynamic and regulatory considerations.* Sports Med 20(4):215-225, 1995.

Lindinger M. *Origins of H+ changes in exercising skeletal muscle.* Can J Appl Physiol 20(3):357-368, 1995.

Loike J. Zalutsky D, Kaback E, Miranda A, Silverstein S. *Extracellular creatine regulates creatine transport in rat and human muscle cells.* Proc Natl Acad Sci 85:807-811, 1988.

Lykken G, Jacob R, Munoz J, Sandstead J. *Mathematical model of creatine metabolism in normal males– cooperation between theory and experiment.* Am. J Clin Nutr 33:2674-85, 1980.

Maughan R. *Creatine supplementation and exercise performance.* Int J Sport Nutrition. 5: 94-101, 1995.

McCann D, Mole P, Caton J. *Phosphocreatine kinetics in humans during exercise and recovery.* Med Sci Sports Exerc 27(3):378-387, 1995.

Mitchell T, AlmadaA, Earnest C. *Creatine reduces blood lipid concentrations in men and women.* FASEB 10(3):3001, 1996.

Radda G. *Control of energy metabolism during muscle contraction.* Diabetes 45(S1):S88-S92, 1996.

Rocic B, Turk Z, Misur I, Vucic M. *Effect of creatine on glycation of albumin in vitro.* Horm Metab Res 27: 511-512, 1995.

Rossiter H, Cannell E, Jakeman P. *The effect of oral creatine supplementation on the 1,000-m performance of competetive rowers.* J Sports Sci: 14: 175-179, 1996.

Sipila I, Rapola J, Simell O, Vannas A. *Supplementary creatine as a treatment for gyrate atrophy of the choroid and retina.* N Engl J Med 304:867-70, 1981.

Smith L, Brunetz M, Chenier T, McCammon M, Houmard J, Franklin M, Israel R. *The effects of static and ballistic stretching on delayed muscle soreness and creatine kinase.* Res Qtrly Exerc Sport 64(1):103-107, 1993.

Soderlund K, Hultman E. *ATP and phosphocreatine changes in single human muscle fibers after intense electrical stimulation.* Am J Physiol 261:E737-741, 1991.

Stockler S, Hanefield F, Frahm J. *Creatine replacement therapy in guanidinoacetate methyltransferase deficiency, a novel inborn error of metabolism.* Lancet 348(9030):789-790, 1996.

Stroud M, Holliman D, Bell D, Green A, Macdonald I, Greenhaff P. *Effect of oral creatine supplementation on respiratory gas exchange and blood lactate accumulation during steady-state incremental treadmill exercise and recovery in man.* Clin Sci 87:707-710, 1994.

Terrillion K, Kolkhorst F, Dolgener F, Joslyn S. *The effect of creatine supplementation on two 700-m maximal running bouts.* Int J Sport Nutr 7(2):138-143, 1997.

Thompson C, Kemp G, Sanderson A, Dixon R, Styles P, Taylor D, Radda G. *Effects of creatine on aerobic and anaerobic metabolism in skeletal muscle in swimmers.* Br J Sports Med 30:222-225, 1996.

Vandenberghe K, Gillis N, Van Leemputte M, Van Hecke P, Vanstapel F, Hespel P. *Caffeine counteracts the ergogenic action of muscle creatine loading.* J Appl Physiol 80(2):452-457, 1996.

Walker J. *Creatine biosynthesis, regulation and function.* Adv Enzymol 50:117-242, 1979.

Walker J. *Metabolic control of creatine biosynthesis: restoration of transamidinase activity following creatine repression.* J Biol Chem 236:493-8, 1960.

ABOUT THE AUTHORS

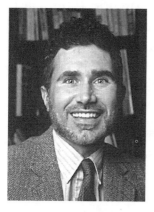 **Ray Sahelian, M.D.,** is a physician certified by the American Board of Family Practice. He obtained a Bachelor of Science degree in nutrition from Drexel University and completed his doctoral training at Thomas Jefferson Medical School, both in Philadelphia. Following graduation he worked for three years as a resident in family medicine at Montgomery Hospital in Norristown, PA, and was involved with all aspects of medical care, including pediatrics, cardiology, obstetrics, oncology, psychiatry, and surgery.

A popular and respected physician and medical writer, Dr. Sahelian is internationally recognized as a moderate voice in the evaluation of leading-edge nutrients and hormones. He has been seen on numerous television programs including *CNN Talk Live, The Maury*

Povich Show, A Current Affair, Extra, Dini Petty Show (Canada), and *Zone Interdite* (France); mentioned by countless major magazines such as *Newsweek, US News and World Report, Cosmopolitan, Modern Medicine, Health,* and *Internal Medicine News;* and quoted in hundreds of newspapers including *USA Today, The Los Angeles Times, The Washington Post, The Miami Herald, The Denver Post, Le Monde* (France), and *Que Pasa* (Chile). His articles have appeared in *Let's Live, Total Health, Healthy and Natural,* and others. Millions of listeners from over 1,000 radio stations nationwide have heard him discuss the latest research on hormones and nutrients.

Dr. Sahelian is the Editor of *Melatonin, DHEA, and Longevity Update,* and a nationally-known lecturer. He is also the author of the highly acclaimed *Be Happier Starting Now,* the bestselling *Melatonin: Nature's Sleeping Pill,* and *DHEA: A Practical Guide.*

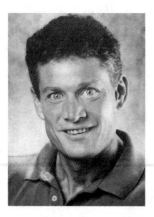

Dave Tuttle has been a writer in the health and fitness field for over a decade. He is a regular contributor to several sports magazines including *Ironman* and *Muscle & Fitness,* and has written about nutrition, exercise and longevity for a variety of journals and newsletters.

His first book, *Forever Natural: How to Excel in Sports Drug-Free,* showed how everyone from varsity athletes to weekend enthusiasts can excel in their chosen sport without the use of steroids. This book has been called "an important addition to sports collections" by *Library Journal*.

Dave Tuttle received a Bachelor of Science degree from Michigan State University and a master's degree from Harvard University. Born and raised in the Midwest, he traveled throughout North and South America before settling in Los Angeles, California, where he currently lives. A lifelong athlete, he has competed in wrestling, gymnastics, and bodybuilding. He started using creatine in 1995, and found the benefits so remarkable that he collaborated with Dr. Sahelian to inform everyone about this exciting supplement.

INDEX

Research in hormone replacement therapy, nutrition, herbs, and longevity is accelerating.

If you wish to keep up with the very latest information on melatonin, DHEA, pregnenolone, estrogen, progesterone, testosterone, growth hormone, other hormones, creatine, glucosamine, herbs, nutrients, and anti-aging medicines, then this is the right newsletter for you. Dr. Sahelian and his staff constantly scan hundreds of new articles published in prestigious journals all over the world and present a balanced interpretation of the important findings. No hype, just the facts. We also discuss advances in the field of anti-aging science and how these advances can be practically applied to improve the quality of our lives. There are no ads in the newsletter and we do not endorse products. All the information is referenced with the latest journal articles.

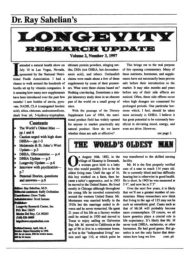

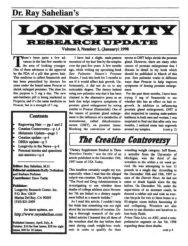

8 PAGES

The newsletter includes interviews with top experts, personal stories of hormone/supplement users, and a question-and-answer column. It is published in January, April, July, and October.

See the last page on how to order.
See web site http://www.raysahelian.com

More than 900,000 copies in print!

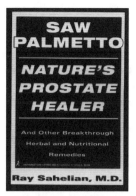

150 pp $5.99   4"x 7"

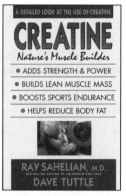

132 pp $9.95 Retail

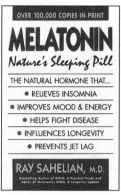

144 pp $9.95 Retail

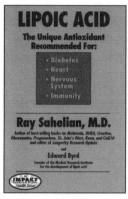

27 pp $3.95 Retail

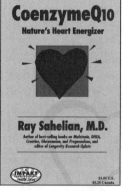

27 pp $3.95 Retail

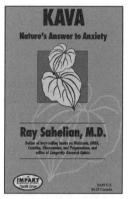

27 pp $3.95 Retail

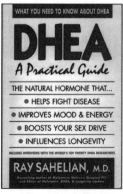

158 pp $9.95 Retail

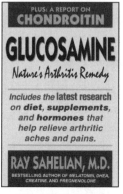

27 pp $3.95 Retail

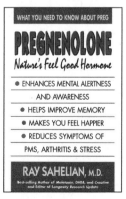

157 pp $9.95 Retail

See web site **http://www.raysahelian.com**. for latest updates. To order by credit card call **310-821-2409** (best times are 9:00 a.m. to 5:00 p.m. Pacific Time, Monday through Friday) or copy/tear this page and mail in your order. Or by credit card thru Email **longrc@aol.com**

Name: _____

Address: _____

City/State/Zip: _____

Telephone: _____ Email: _____

❑ 4 issues Longevity Research Update . . . .$16.00____
❑ 8 issues of Longevity Research Update . . . .$28.00____
❑ 16 issues of Longevity Research Update . . . .$48.00____

Newsletters began in Jan. 1996 and are published quarterly (January, April, July, October). Back issues are $1.00 each. $ _____

_____ copies *Creatine: Nature's Muscle Builder* . . . .*$9.95*_____
_____ copies *DHEA: A Practical Guide* . . . .*$9.95*_____
_____ copies *Melatonin: Nature's Sleeping Pill* . . . .*$9.95*_____
_____ copies *Pregnenolone: Nature's Feel Good Hormone* . . . .*$9.95*_____
_____ copies *Glucosamine: Nature's Arthritis Remedy* . . . .*$3.95*_____
_____ copies *Kava: Nature's Answer to Anxiety* . . . .*$3.95*_____
_____ copies *CoQ10: Nature's Heart Energizer* . . . .*$3.95*_____
_____ copies *Lipoic Acid: The Unique Antioxidant* . . . .*$3.95*_____
_____ copies *Saw Palmetto: Nature's Prostate Healer* . . . .*$5.99*_____
Books on Stevia, 5-HTP, and other topics coming soon. Call for details.

No shipping charge for books mailed to US or Canada.
Shipping (airmail) for overseas: add $7.00 for first book,
$3.00 for each additional book, and 70¢ for each newsletter   _____
Tax on books shipped to California addresses is 8%   _____

Total: $_____

Books and newsletters are shipped promptly.

Please send a check for the total amount to:
Longevity Research Center, Inc.
P. O. Box 12619
Marina Del Rey, CA 90295

Credit Card #_____ Exp. _____
We accept Visa, MC, AE, Diners Club, Carte Blanche, and JCB.

Healthy Habits

are easy to come by—

IF YOU KNOW WHERE TO LOOK!

Get the latest information on:
- better health • diet & weight loss
- the latest nutritional supplements
- herbal healing • homeopathy and more

COMPLETE AND RETURN THIS CARD RIGHT AWAY!

Where did you purchase this book?
- ❑ bookstore
- ❑ health food store
- ❑ pharmacy
- ❑ supermarket
- ❑ other (please specify)_____

Name_____

Street Address_____

City_____State_____Zip_____

RECEIVE A FREE COPY OF AVERY'S HEALTH CATALOG

GIVE ONE TO A FRIEND . . .

Healthy Habits

are easy to come by—

IF YOU KNOW WHERE TO LOOK!

Get the latest information on:
- better health • diet & weight loss
- the latest nutritional supplements
- herbal healing • homeopathy and more

COMPLETE AND RETURN THIS CARD RIGHT AWAY!

Where did you purchase this book?
- ❑ bookstore
- ❑ health food store
- ❑ pharmacy
- ❑ supermarket
- ❑ other (please specify)_____

Name_____

Street Address_____

City_____State_____Zip_____

RECEIVE A FREE COPY OF AVERY'S HEALTH CATALOG

PLACE
STAMP
HERE

Avery Publishing Group
120 Old Broadway
Garden City Park, NY 11040

I..II...III....I..III....I.I.II.....II.I.I...II.I

PLACE
STAMP
HERE

Avery Publishing Group
120 Old Broadway
Garden City Park, NY 11040

I..II...III....I..III....I.I.II.....II.I.I...II.I